There are many pieces to the mental wellness puzzle, and in their second cookbook, certified nutritionists Tamara Green and Sarah Grossman focus on one element that you can control: food. By taking you through the latest science, in clear, digestible bites, they provide key takeaways that you can implement into your daily life to help you support your mood through food. Inside, you'll discover how to:

Understand the Basics: Learn how to make better food choices that will support your mental health—without completely cutting out sweets or grasping for other "quick-fix" solutions.

Empower Yourself: At a glance, each recipe identifies the mood and nutrient benefits you may experience with that specific dish, including balancing blood sugar, providing protein, delivering healthy fats, supplying fiber, and more.

Take Action: Apply this knowledge to your daily meal planning with over 100 recipes spanning Breakfasts, Snacks, Mains, Sides, Desserts, and Drinks.

Eat for Your Mood: Depending on your needs, snack on Easy Seedy Flax Crackers to help balance blood sugar and enhance focus; enjoy Ribboned Carrot Slaw with Miso Sesame Vinaigrette to help ease anxiety by supporting gut health; and feast on Crispy Turmeric Chicken Thighs for a protein-rich meal to create feel-good neurotransmitters.

With mental health at the forefront of so many people's minds, exploring the relationship between brain and gut health has never been more important. With *Good Food, Good Mood* as your guide, you'll gain the confidence and knowledge needed to make the best choices for your mental well-being—and overall health—today and long into the future.

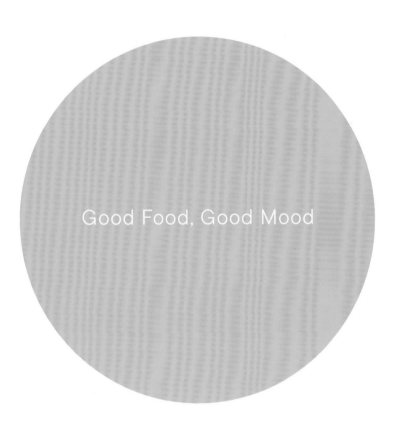

Good Food, Good Mood

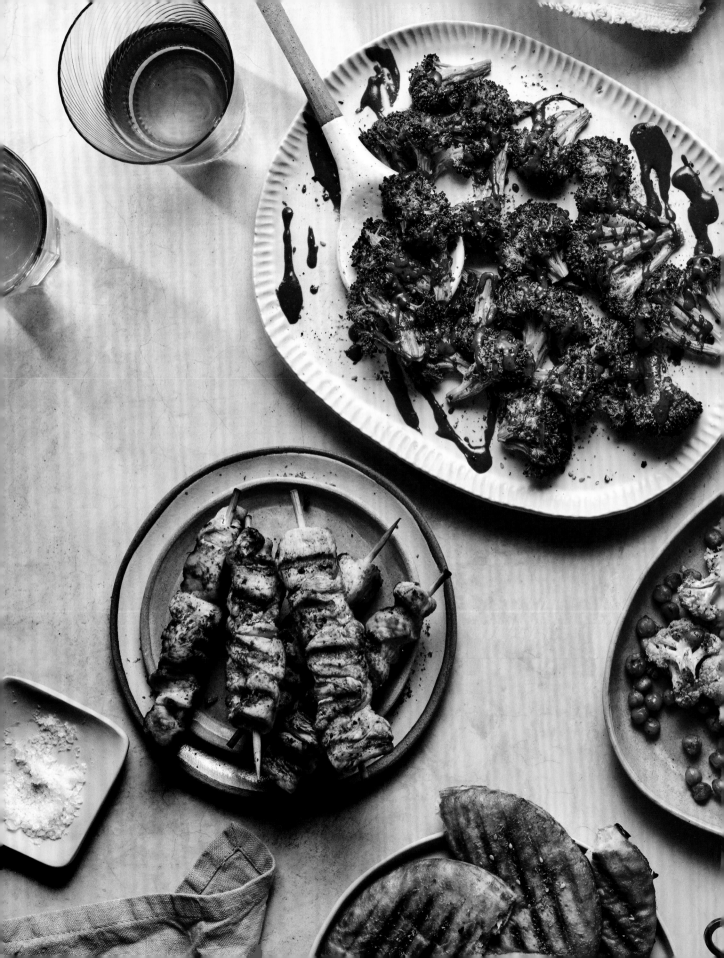

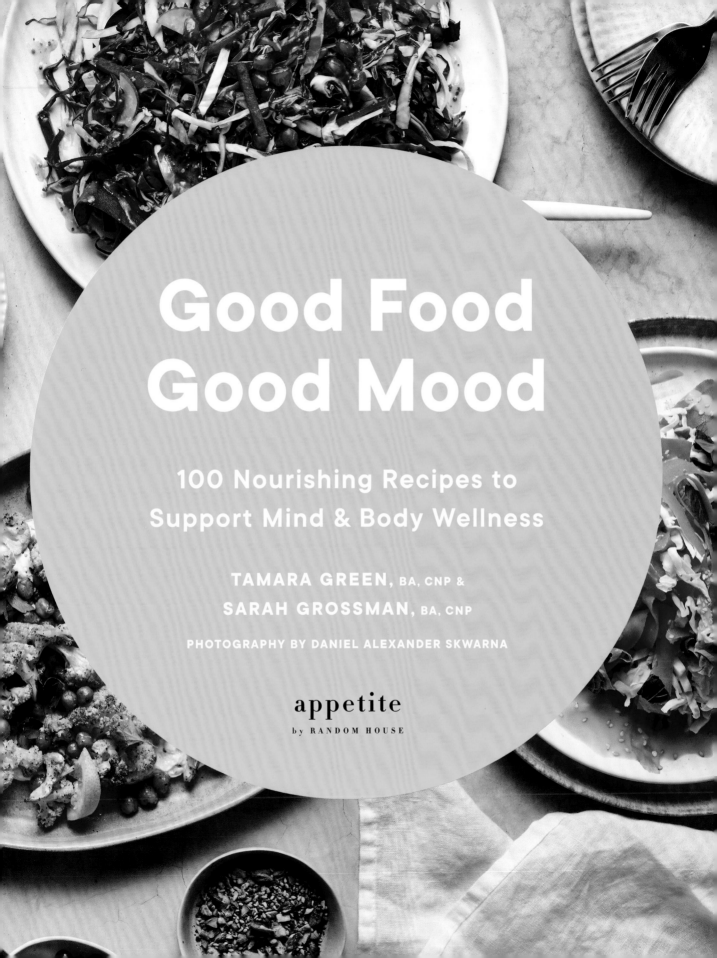

Good Food Good Mood

100 Nourishing Recipes to Support Mind & Body Wellness

TAMARA GREEN, BA, CNP &
SARAH GROSSMAN, BA, CNP

PHOTOGRAPHY BY DANIEL ALEXANDER SKWARNA

appetite
by RANDOM HOUSE

Appetite by Random House® and colophon are registered trademarks of Penguin Random House LLC.

This publication contains the opinions and ideas of its authors. It is intended to provide helpful and informative material on the subjects addressed in the publication. It is sold with the understanding that the author and publisher are not engaged in rendering medical, health, or any kind of personal professional services. Nutritional and other needs vary depending on age, sex, and health status. If you suspect that you have a serious medical problem, the authors strongly urge you to consult your medical or health professional for treatment.

Library and Archives Canada Cataloguing in Publication is available upon request.

ISBN: 978-0-525-61198-1
eBook ISBN: 978-0-525-61199-8

Cover and book design: Talia Abramson
Cover and interior food photography: Daniel Alexander Skwarna
Author photos: Shannon Laliberte
Food styling: Sarah Grossman and Tamara Green
Prop styling: Rayna Schwartz
Printed in China

Published in Canada by Appetite by Random House®,
a division of Penguin Random House Canada Limited.

www.penguinrandomhouse.ca

10 9 8 7 6 5 4 3 2 1

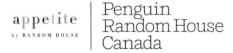

To our community: clients, readers, friends, and family, we hope this book inspires you to cook delicious food, eat well, and feel really good.

Daniel, Lumi, Bram, Jackson, and Reese, we love you.

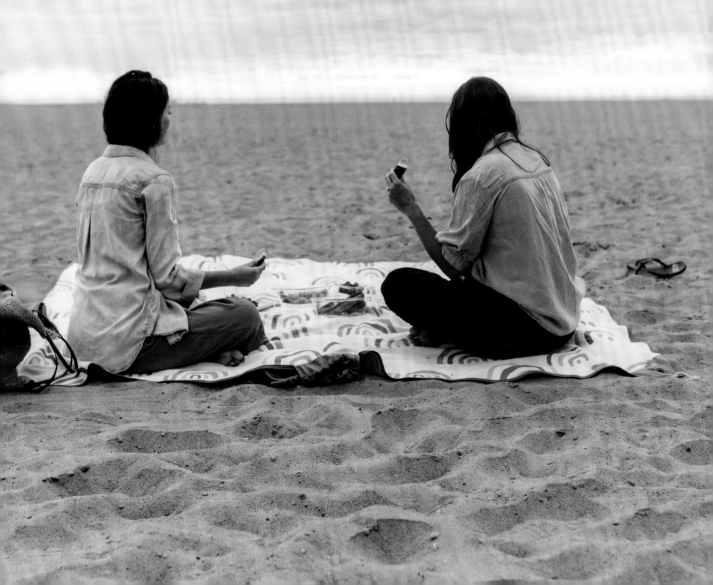

Contents

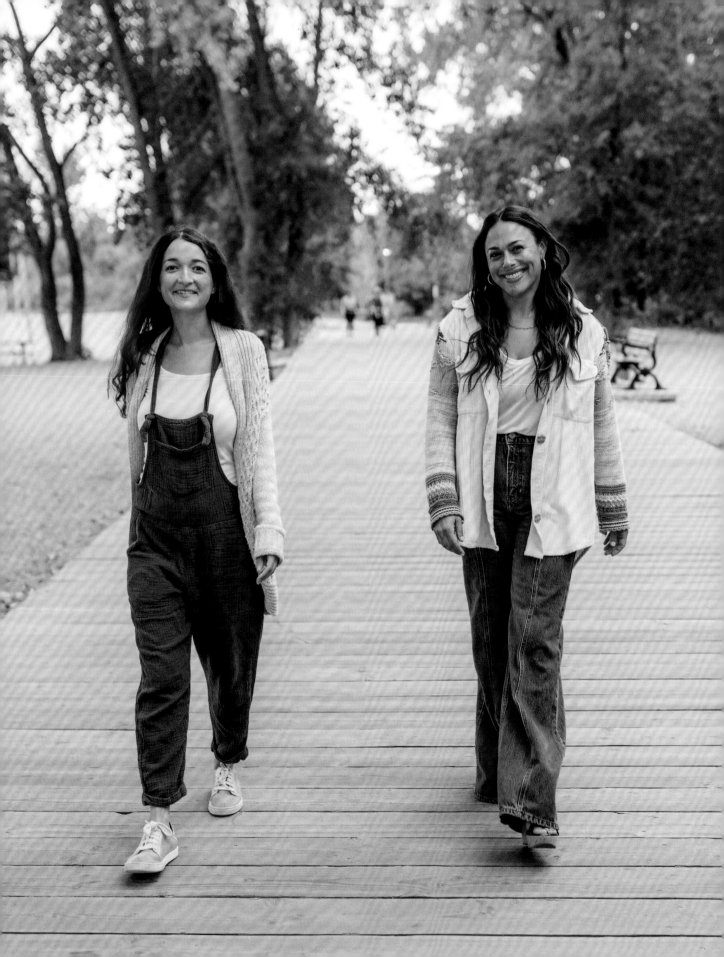

Can What You Eat Actually Improve Your Mood?

The short answer is: yes!

When we set out to create a cookbook about food and mood, we were inspired to write all about the "happiness" diet. Here's what happened instead: we were thrust into a pandemic (like everyone else) while working and parenting, and fell into a hole of deep sadness, grief, loss, loneliness, anxiety, depression, and confusion. It felt so ironic that we were writing a cookbook on how to elevate one's mental health while ours was slowly suffering.

The truth is, together, our mental health, brain health, and mood is a composite of many things—not just one. It's made up of diet, movement, stress-releasing practices, quality sleep, connection with others, physical safety, community, strong sense of self, past experiences, self-compassion, genetics, and sometimes medication, therapy, and supplements.

We wanted to show our readers how to become the happiest versions of themselves all through a simple shift in diet. *Ta-da! Get those jazz hands out, because here is your before-and-after happiness picture!* While there is a big element of truth to this—food absolutely impacts mood and our mental well-being—what we learned is that it's not a linear process, nor is it human to be happy all the time.

If we hadn't been mindful of the food we were eating and the thoughts we were thinking during this time, if we hadn't been committed to balancing our blood sugar (we'll explain what this means shortly), eating colorful vegetables, getting enough protein, and enjoying healthy sweets, then that small hole we were in would have become a deep, gaping, dark crevasse. There are many pieces to the mental wellness puzzle, and in this book our focus is on food.

Using food as a way to improve mental health and mood is somewhat new. For a large part of history, including in the last few decades, mental health wasn't even really acknowledged as being a thing. It was something elusive; we couldn't point to it and say "There it is!" like doctors would with a broken bone or a cluster of cancer cells. Nonetheless, nowadays, more people worldwide suffer from depression than from any other health issue, and according to the World Health Organization, 280 million people live with depression. In addition to that, 1 in 13 people world-wide suffer from an anxiety disorder, with 40 million Americans living with some type of anxiety every year.[1]

Many factors contribute to the burden on our mental health, whether it be war and violence, climate change and natural disasters, everyday personal stressors like work, raising a family, losing a loved one, or dealing with a health crisis . . . the list goes on and on. But we'd be remiss not to mention how much the COVID-19 pandemic has impacted the global collective's mental health. In the US alone, nearly one in five Americans said their mental health was worse in 2020 than it was in 2019, and the American Psychological Association has stated we are facing a mental health crisis.[2] Although many of our lives have gone back to "normal" the impact of the pandemic still lingers.

Now more than ever, we see how important it is that people have access to information that can help them empower their mental well-being. And this is exactly what we intend to do with this cookbook. What we've learned from all our research—reviewing studies, working with clients, using ourselves as test subjects—is that the nutrients we eat greatly impact all areas of the body: our gut microbes, our hormones, our neurotransmitters, our vitamin and mineral stores, our nervous system, and so much more. And this impact has a direct effect on the thoughts we think, the feelings we experience, the amount of energy we have, and, truly, our overall mental well-being. So yes, what we eat can actually make us feel better and improve our mood.

BUT WHO ARE WE TO TELL YOU THAT YOUR DIET CAN DO ALL THIS?

We're certified nutritionists and wellness chefs. But before we get into that, first we'd like to tell you our personal stories about how our diets greatly influenced our own mental health.

Tamara: I grew up as a very anxious kid—riddled with fear, crippled with stomach aches and a picky-eating complex. I had anxiety about everything. I was anxious my parents wouldn't be there to pick me up from the camp bus. I was terrified of my third-grade teacher, Ms. Weinback, who once told me that her "bark was much worse than her bite" (I sometimes feel like I missed the third grade entirely because I was too scared to go). I was nervous about going on planes, taking tests, having sleepovers with friends, and going to extracurricular activities like gymnastics.

I was also a very picky eater—not for lack of trying from my parents—and stuck to a strict hamburger-fries-pizza-only diet that led to tummy aches, vomiting, and frequent trips to the bathroom. I was given a blanket diagnosis of irritable bowel syndrome (IBS) and sent on my way with no direction. I learned only years later that some of my childhood anxiety may have been exacerbated by or connected to my poor eating habits and digestive issues. Today, I'm the parent of a picky eater, and I can understand how challenging it is to get selective eaters to eat, let alone try new foods.

Even if my parents had known about the connection between anxiety and nutrition back then, they would have needed a lot more tools to help me change my diet. At the time, their solution was to send me to a child psychologist. I remember lying down on the couch in Dr. Gerald Buttons' office, practicing meditation, visualization, and breathing (before these types of practices were in vogue). Like many childhood anxieties, mine began to dissipate as I got older, thanks in part to the tools Dr. Buttons taught me—until they reared their ugly head when I became pregnant with my first child. I would wake up at 3 a.m. in pools of sweat, crying uncontrollably, feeling the heaviest of weights on my chest, and could not be consoled. My old childhood anxieties had come back, except this time it wasn't about whether I was going to let my gymnastics team down, it was about how I was going to function as a parent: *What if something happens to my husband? How do I work and parent as an entrepreneur? What the heck am I doing?*

My obstetrician was a bit concerned about me and so sent me to a psychiatrist. Many people talk about postpartum depression, but prenatal depression and anxiety are also very real, though often left out of the conversation. The psychiatrist told me medication wouldn't help me. Luckily, I had the wherewithal to seek out help on my own and build a community of support. My diet was already quite healthy, but over time I really honed in on what I was eating, paying special attention to my blood sugar and its role in my mental well-being. The whole pregnancy was not without its mental challenges, but gathering various tools along the way, especially when it came to my diet, helped ease a lot of my anxious feelings by the time I gave birth.

Now, in the sandwich generation, I'm entering a new phase of life as I parent young kids and also support my mom through a mental health crisis she is facing. It truly does take a village and a whole toolbox to support mental wellness, and food is one of the essentials inside that toolbox. I know that when I experience mental dips and dark lows, I can see a connection between those feelings and what I ate days prior. For me, eating well—which involves keeping my blood sugar steady, getting lots of colorful veggies, and ensuring I have protein at every meal—is a major component of keeping my mood balanced and maintaining my emotional health.

Sarah: As a kid, I set my heart on becoming a professional ballerina. It was my everything. I practiced ballet every day—after school I was off to dance class, and every summer I spent months at intensive ballet camps. I was constantly worried about my body and whether I was good enough to compete. Was I truly trying hard enough? Would I fit in? There were a million things to worry about. I often wonder if my high internal stress load as a young adult was a direct result of those crazy-intense years— and if that formative experience impacts how I handle stress and anxiety as an adult.

My worries were also body-based. I spent most of my twenties terrified of my period. Every month I'd end up in bed, depressed and lonely. I felt awful about myself, and before I came to understand why, I felt that something was really wrong with me. Eventually, I learned I had endometriosis. Knowing this helped me understand the physical "why," but it didn't solve how I felt emotionally and mentally.

There are so many things that helped me get a better handle on my physical and mental well-being, including acupuncture, massage, naturopathic medicine, movement, community and friends, time in nature, and therapy. But one other essential component was food. I had known for a long time that what I ate impacted my physical health, but I didn't always pay attention to how it impacted my mood. After finding out about the endometriosis, I wanted to feel better emotionally and get a handle on my anxiety and stress. I found that what I ate made a huge difference. I needed good proteins and healthy fats in my meals and snacks to feel balanced and have energy. When I got hungry and my blood sugar dropped, I didn't feel well. I realized that I lost focus and became even more anxious. It all made sense—it was more difficult to self-regulate my emotions if physically I didn't feel well.

Fast-forward to the present and I still worry about many areas of my life. That didn't just go away when I stopped dancing. It shows up in different ways as an adult: negative self-talk about my body, worrying about my daughter in the middle of the night, or catastrophizing that something awful will happen to my husband because he has type 1 diabetes. It's a lot to handle the everyday stresses of work and parenting, along with the worries about my parents' mental health as they get older. But making sure I have nourishing, delicious food available at home, and prioritizing time to eat balanced meals and snacks, makes a world of a difference in how I feel—both emotionally and mentally—each day.

I know how challenging it all can be, not just for myself but for some of my closest family members and friends—some days we're great at implementing the things that we know help us feel better, and other days not so much. Making space for the practices that support our mental well-being and mood is an ongoing process, and I hope this book can be part of an overall strategy that helps you. I'm so happy you've found our cookbook!

HOW WE HELP OUR CLIENTS (AND NOW, YOU!)

We graduated from the Institute of Holistic Nutrition, in Toronto, in 2010 and opened our company, The Living Kitchen, that same year. One of our first jobs was teaching cooking classes to out-patients at the Canadian Mental Health Association, showing how impactful healthy food can be on one's mental health, while also making it accessible and delicious. We eventually started a meal-delivery service and then a private-chef service, and we counseled people on how to eat to feel the best they could, always meeting them where they were at. Our clients ranged from celebrities in town filming movies to couples looking for easy dinners, families with picky eaters, women experiencing anxiety from struggling with infertility or postpartum depression, cancer patients and their caregivers, people with dementia and Alzheimer's, CEOs recovering from burnout, and people experiencing debilitating digestive issues. Here's what we learned: when someone is physically suffering, they are most likely suffering mentally too (and vice versa). Our goal for our clients (and ourselves) has been the same since the beginning: feed people good, nutritious food so they can feel as best as possible, both physically and mentally.

WHAT'S NEXT

In the coming chapters, we put our goal into practice. We'll teach you how the foods you eat have a direct impact on your mental health and mood by way of feeding the microbes in your gut, building neurotransmitters (feel-good chemicals), supporting your nervous system, and balancing your blood sugar, among other ways. But once you know all this info, how do you implement it? Don't worry; we'll help you put it into practice on page 35. And then, of course, perhaps our favorite part: the recipes. Let the science-backed information, combined with the gorgeous food photos and recipes, inspire you to cook, eat, and (hopefully) improve your mood.

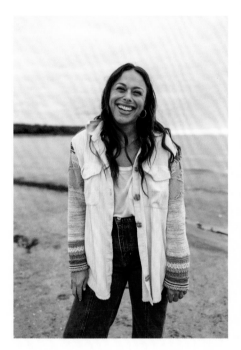

Tamara

Sarah

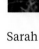

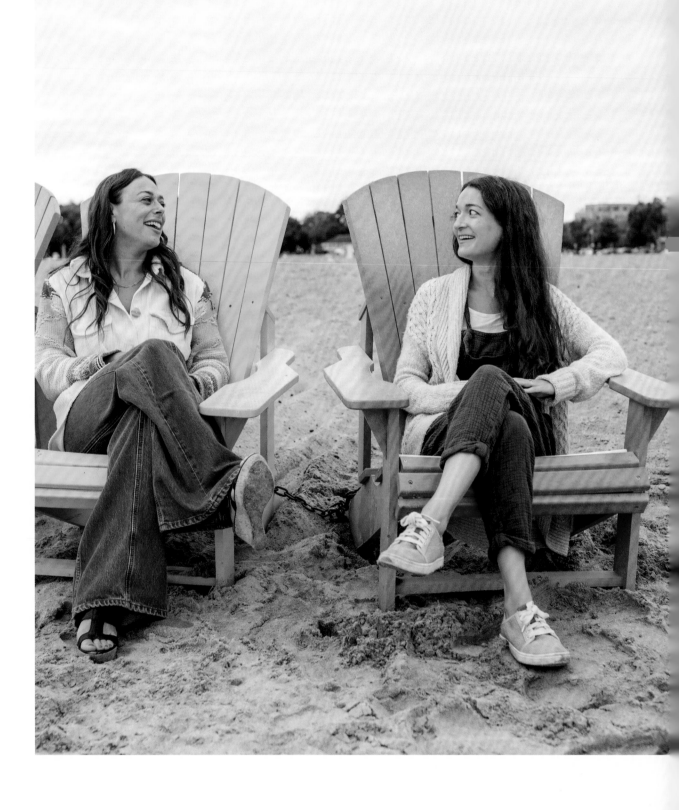

Hi Brain, It's Me, Gut . . . We Need to Talk

When we think about our body, we often picture it in separate parts. We have lungs, a heart, a liver, kidneys all taking up space inside our body. Yet, we forget how inter-connected these parts of our body are and the incredible dance they do daily to keep us upright and functioning—living! Inside of these magical bodies of ours is a flurry of activity and communication as every single part of us is working hard to keep a homeostatic balance. Two organs in constant communication are our brain and our gut. By "gut" we mean the gastrointestinal/digestive tract—everything from the esophagus to the rectum.

The gut and brain talk to each other about enzymes, digestion, immune cells, hormones, heart rate, behavior, emotions, and memory. They're talking about that scary meeting you have coming up with your boss, parallel parking your car in a tight spot while someone waits behind you, that exciting date you're going on, your upcoming public speaking event in front of a huge audience, and maybe even an awful email you just received.

The gut and brain are inextricably linked, which is why the gut is referred to as the "second brain." It's lined with millions and millions of neurons (cells that send and receive info to and from the nervous system and brain). Another reason for its nick-name is that certain neurotransmitters (aka chemical messengers), such as serotonin (the happy chemical), dopamine (the pleasure chemical), and GABA (the calming chemical), are largely produced in the gut.

HOW DO YOUR BRAIN AND GUT ACTUALLY TALK TO EACH OTHER?

The most direct route between the gut and the brain is through the vagus nerve. In Latin, *vagus* means *wanderer*, and it's a suitable name for this nerve that "wanders" from the brain throughout the body, picking up lots of key information about the inner organs—those of the digestive system, plus the liver, heart, and lungs—and delivering this information back to the brain. This is one of the ways the brain knows what's going on in the body. The brain processes the information it's given and then gives its response.[3] For example, if a pathogen (in the form of food poisoning) has infiltrated the gut, the gut sounds the alarm to the brain via the vagus nerve, the brain then responds by sending signals to get the toxin out of the body immediately, the vomit valve opens . . . and you know the rest!

Many people experience physical sensations of anxiety, stress, sadness, depression, excitement, nervousness, and extreme joy in the form of things like heart palpitations, sudden or frequent bowel movements, constipation, diarrhea, nausea, vomiting, tremors, shakiness, appetite loss, or appetite gain. This has to do with the wandering vagus nerve sending signals throughout the body, especially between the gut and the brain.

WHEN THE GUT SUFFERS, SO DOES THE BRAIN

It's only been in the last decade or so that research has found a connection between mental health and the gut. People who experience chronic stress, anxiety, depression, and other mental health challenges often also experience inflammatory bowel disease (Crohn's disease or ulcerative colitis), food intolerances, irritable bowel syndrome, gut inflammation, and dysbiosis (an imbalance of bacteria in your gut).[4]

Our body is a complex, interconnected system, and when something happens in one area, it doesn't necessarily stay only there. For instance, if your gut is inflamed and irritated, it may impact the health of your gut bacteria and communication signaling with the brain. This can go on to disrupt brain neurochemistry, increase vulnerability to anxiety and depression and impact behavior. If your brain senses stress, it diverts energy away from the gut, which may damage the gut over time, especially if the stress is chronic, and this eventually can contribute to serious digestive problems.

LET'S TELL YOU ABOUT OUR CLIENT JASON

Jason suffered from severe digestive issues for years and years. He was working a 70-plus-hour workweek, traveled a ton, and scarfed down most meals in minutes while eating them on the go; lately, his appetite had been waning. To say he was stressed is an understatement—he was overwhelmed, tired, and anxious. His symptoms were getting so bad he had lost 40 pounds, and this weight loss made him even more anxious. When we started working together, we had to take small steps—actually, baby steps—to help dig him out of the stress hole he was sinking into. Our first focus was slowly revamping his diet and helping him prioritize himself, because at this rate, he was going to crash and burn. As we continually helped him choose more gut-friendly foods—which we'll tell you about soon—his digestion started to improve and so did his mood. He started putting weight back on, feeling more like himself, and even feeling . . . happier. It's incredible what diet and self-care can do, especially when paired together.

MEET OUR FRIENDS AND YOURS: THE MICROBES

Look down at your hands. Yes, right now. Take a good look. Even though you can't see them, at this very moment, your hands are covered in bacteria—actually, your whole body is! *Inside* our bodies, there is one place in particular that houses trillions of bacteria, and that's your gut—mainly your colon. Some scientists like to say that we are more bacteria than we are human.

The gut microbiome is often referred to as an ecosystem or a rainforest because it has a diverse population of microbes like bacteria, archaea, fungi, viruses, and parasites—which live together, rely on each other, and work symbiotically. Your microbiome is unique to you, just like your thumbprint is. No one else in this world has an identical one—not even your identical twin, if you have one—and the microbes that colonize the gut are there because of genetics, where you live in the world, your diet, current or past illnesses, antibiotic use, medication, supplementation, stress, traumatic events, the people you live with, and even your pets.

How Your Microbes Impact Your Mood

So, what do these microbes have to do with happiness, joy, anxiety, depression, sadness, stress, and brain fog? A lot! Research has found a strong association between microbiome function and mental well-being.[5] First, those teeny, tiny microbes have a lot to do. Giulia Enders, the author of *Gut*, writes: "Microbes crack open indigestible foodstuffs for us [think: fiber], supply the gut with energy, manufacture vitamins [like B_{12}], break down toxins and medications, and train our immune system."[6]

Another one of their jobs is to produce and regulate neurotransmitters (as discussed on page 24). You know, the ones responsible for happiness, motivation, focus, learning, memory, reward, pleasure, and neuroplasticity. For these to be made and regulated, you need healthy, functioning, diverse gut microbes, but you also need nutrients from food, which act as building blocks for the neurotransmitters. **Your diet and what you eat directly influences the microbes in your gut.**

Once we feed microbes the food they love (ahem, fiber), they ferment it to create metabolites (small particles that food gets broken down into), one of them being butyrate. Butyrate and its friends have many jobs, like keeping the lining of the gut strong and dampening inflammation—this is key for immunity. When we lack butyrate and have an imbalance of harmful gut microbes, the lining of the gut can become inflamed or permeable. Inflammatory sirens will then go off in the body and brain, influencing brain function and possibly leading to anxiety, depression, and memory loss.[7]

Our friends—the microbes—also influence our emotions and behavior by stimulating and activating the vagus nerve (remember, the wandering nerve that connects the brain with the gut and a number of other significant organs).[8]

A DIVERSE GUT IS A HEALTHY GUT

Although we each have our own unique microbiome, it can still share similarities with others. A healthy gut microbiome is one that has a diverse population of microbes. Scientists have found that people are more likely to suffer from depression if their gut is missing some of the good strains of bacteria.[9] The American Gut Project looked at over fifteen thousand stool samples from 11,335 human participants, mainly from the US and the UK.[10] They found that those who identified as having depression, schizophrenia, PTSD, and bipolar disorder had a similar gut makeup compared with those who didn't identify as having these disorders.[11] Similarly, the Flemish Gut Flora Project examined stool from one thousand participants and found that those who experienced depression were missing the same two microbial strains in their gut and had a much less diverse microbe population, especially compared with people who identified as having a high quality of life.[12]

Having a healthy, diverse gut is integral to mood, mental health, and overall well-being, but what does a healthy gut actually look like, and how do you get one? In the next chapter, we'll share all those details.

THE BIG TAKEAWAYS

- The gut and brain talk to each other via the vagus nerve, and the gut is often referred to as the "second brain."
- If the gut is inflamed or irritated from a digestive issue or excessive stress, this impacts communication between it and the brain.
- You have over 100 trillion microbes in your gut; these have many jobs, like producing and regulating neurotransmitters (chemical messengers responsible for happiness, motivation, focus, and feeling calm).
- Microbes need fiber to flourish.
- People with a more diverse gut tend to have a higher quality of life.

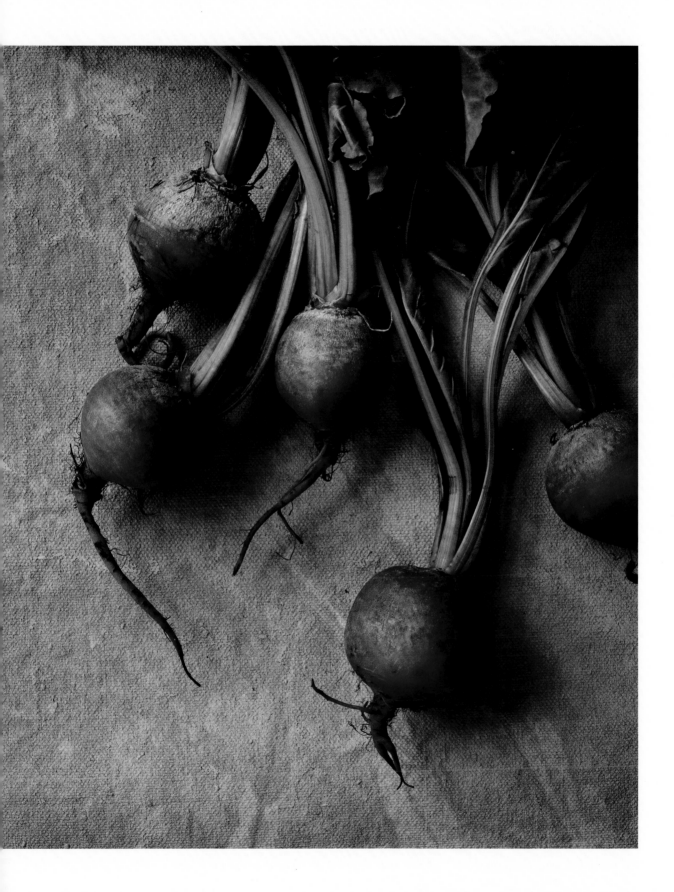

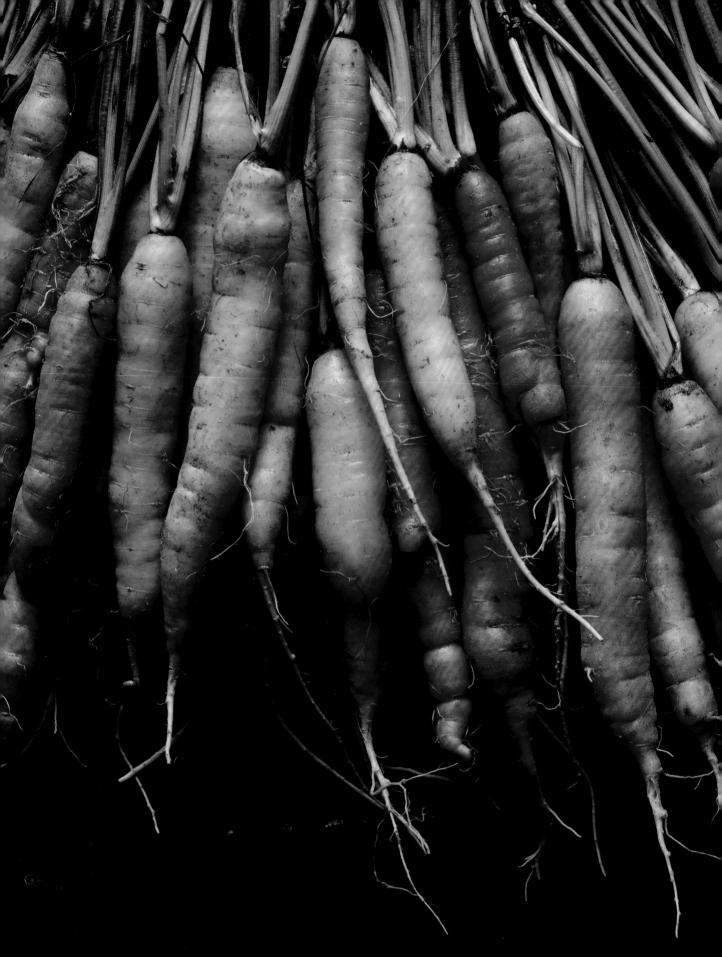

Foods That Support Mood

Now that you know that your gut and brain are deeply connected, and that food plays a significant role in strengthening this connection, it's time to learn how to ensure you create or maintain a diverse, flourishing gut to support your mood and mental health. We'll also give you the lowdown on integral nutrients to eat to help achieve a calm, focused, and steady mind.

First, here's what you need to know: what you eat either feeds beneficial bacteria, starves bacteria, or feeds harmful pathogens or bacteria. The good guys in your gut are always trying to outcompete the bad, and the number one nutrient that helps the good guys succeed in their battle is fiber.

FIBER

When you hear the word "fiber," you may immediately think of the 1990s versions of dry, brown fiber-enriched cereal or powdered fiber supplements you need to chug with water. To be clear, that is *not* what we're talking about here. The best place to find fiber is directly at the source: plants, including legumes, nuts, seeds, whole grains, vegetables, and fruits.

For many years, people just thought fiber kept you regular. But it's got a few more jobs than that, and one of the most important ones is to feed the good bacteria in your gut, helping maintain the delicate balance between all the hundreds of trillions of microorganisms that live there. The healthy bacteria eat the fiber and from it make byproducts that help seal the gut lining, strengthen communication between the gut and brain, synthesize some vitamins (even though we get lots of vitamins from food, some are also manufactured by bacteria in the gut, like vitamins K and B_{12}), and reduce inflammation; this all has a major impact on the immune system and mood regulation.[13] You absolutely need fiber to have a healthy gut microbiome.

How Much Fiber Do You Need?

Increasing your fiber, even over a short period, makes a big difference. In a small study out of University of California Irvine, participants ate between 40 and 50 grams of fiber per day for two weeks.[14] To give you some context, most people only eat about 10 to 15 grams of fiber daily. Researchers found that after this two-week high-fiber period, the composition of participants' gut microbiomes were altered significantly. It's never too late to start eating your fiber!

The general recommendation for fiber intake is about 25 grams of fiber per day. Ideally, you're getting closer to 40 grams or even 50 grams, but this may take some time to work up to. If you increase it too quickly, you may notice some unwanted wind or bloating, so be mindful of increasing your intake at your own speed. Sometimes it's hard to know how much fiber you're actually eating, so we have a handy chart below, that highlights the amount of fiber per serving in a variety of plant foods.

Can You Eat 30-Plus Different Plants a Week?

Another great way to rack up your fiber points is by counting your plants and seeing if you can eat 30 types of plants a week. The American Gut Project—remember, its researchers looked at over fifteen thousand stool samples (page 10)—found something interesting when inspecting all that poo: that those who ate 30 or more types of plants per week had the most diverse population of microbes in their gut, especially compared with those who ate only 10 or fewer types of plants per week.[15] Remember, *all* plants count; this isn't limited to fruits and vegetables.

Sources of Fiber

FOOD SOURCE	AMOUNT OF FIBER (g)
1 apple with skin	4.5
1 cup black beans	12
1 cup blueberries	4
½ cup cooked broccoli	2.5
1 cup brown rice	4
1 cup cooked Brussels sprouts	4
½ cup cooked carrots	2.5
½ cup cooked cauliflower	1.7
1 Tbsp chia seeds	4
1 cup chickpeas	10
1 Tbsp whole flaxseeds	2
½ cup cooked green beans	2

FOOD SOURCE	AMOUNT OF FIBER (g)
3 Tbsp hemp seeds	2
1 cup kidney beans	10
1 cup lentils	16
1 cup navy beans	19
1 cup northern white beans	16
1 pear with skin	5.5
½ cup cooked pumpkin	5
1 cup quinoa	5
1 cup raspberries	8
½ cup cooked spinach	2.2
½ cup cooked squash	3
1 cup strawberries	3
½ cup sweet potato	3
1 Tbsp tahini	1.4

Fiber and Blood Sugar

Fiber plays an enormous role in blood sugar balance. A topic we are passionate about (in the next chapter, we'll try to get you passionate about it too!). Fiber is structurally complex, so the body takes a while to break it down, which in turn slows blood sugar from spiking (a very good thing). Balanced blood sugar is integral to a stable, focused, and steady mood (among many, many other things).

FERMENTED FOODS AND PROBIOTICS

How Food Ferments

Many cultures have some form of fermented food, and it often but not always begins with a vegetable, a bit of water, some salt, and sometimes a "starter" (consisting of good bacteria), typically in a glass jar set out at room temperature. The good bacteria work to break down the sugars in the food, eventually creating lactic acid, which is what gives many of these foods their tangy, often sour, taste—and also kills off bad bacteria that would make you sick if you were to consume it. The bacteria responsible for transforming these foods into fermented versions of themselves are the same bacteria you often find in a bottle of probiotics, like *Lactobacillus* and *Bifidobacterium*. Fermented foods are a wonderful source of these good strains of bacteria that multiply during the fermentation process.

The Benefits of Probiotics

Probiotics are live microorganisms that provide health benefits to the person consuming them. People have questioned if the probiotics in these fermented foods could survive the journey from mouth to colon, making it there alive. A team of Stanford University researchers have confirmed they can, and found that after just a few weeks of eating a diet rich in fermented foods, microbe diversity in the gut increased and inflammatory markers decreased.[16] This is a big deal—microbial diversity has been connected with a higher quality of life and has influence over the immune system and mental health, like helping to alleviate depression.[17]

Getting Fermented Foods into Your Diet

While some favorite foods—chocolate, sourdough bread, wine, and cheese—are fermented, it's important to understand that some ferments offer more health benefits to their host (you!) than others. The good news is that, nowadays, it's easy to eat those nutritious fermented foods, since they're readily available at many grocery stores. It's best to choose the ferments found in the refrigerator section of your supermarket, as most shelf-stable ferments use vinegar, which kills the delicate bacteria we're hoping will populate the gut. It's not just yogurt that's a great option, but also sauerkraut, kimchi, and lacto-fermented pickles. All are excellent additions to salads or served on the side of a meal.

Other great ferments include:
- **Kefir:** Similar to yogurt but thinner, it can be used in smoothies or sipped by the glass.
- **Miso and tempeh:** These fermented soy foods are savory, salty, and bring an umami flavor to cooking. Tempeh can be used to replace tofu, and miso works well in sauces and dressings.
- **Kombucha:** This fizzy fermented tea is a delicious option, but seek out low-sugar varieties.

How Much Fermented Food Should You Eat?

Ideally, you should eat 1–3 servings of fermented foods a day, though we know this isn't always possible. One serving looks like:
- ½–1 cup yogurt
- 2 tablespoons sauerkraut or kimchi
- ¼–½ cup kefir
- 1 cup kombucha
- 3 oz of tempeh
- 1 Tbsp miso in soup, or dressing

PREBIOTICS AND RESISTANT STARCHES

Many people have heard of probiotics, but not everyone has heard of *prebiotics*. Prebiotics feed the healthy bacteria (the probiotics) in your gut. Prebiotics are found in plant fibers in asparagus, onions, garlic, endive, Jerusalem artichokes, chia seeds, unripe green bananas, mushrooms, leeks, oats, and rye (we have plenty of recipes that include these ingredients in this book!). Your body can't digest these prebiotics, so they pass right on through to become grub for your gut microbes.[18]

Resistant starches (starches that resist digestion) are considered prebiotics too. These are found in cooked and cooled potatoes, rice, lentils, chickpeas, and black beans, among other foods. When these foods are cooked and then cooled, their chemical makeup changes; they then bypass digestion in your small intestine, creating a feast for your microbes in your large intestine (colon). Prebiotics fuel *only* the helpful microbes, which ultimately helps the good guys grow and flourish.[19] The harmful bacteria can't process prebiotics, so they lose out.[20]

How Much Prebiotic Food Should You Eat?

There is no official guideline for how many prebiotics to eat per day, but studies suggest that if you're meeting fiber goals (a minimum 25 grams of fiber per day), you're likely eating enough. Although all prebiotics are considered fiber, not all fiber

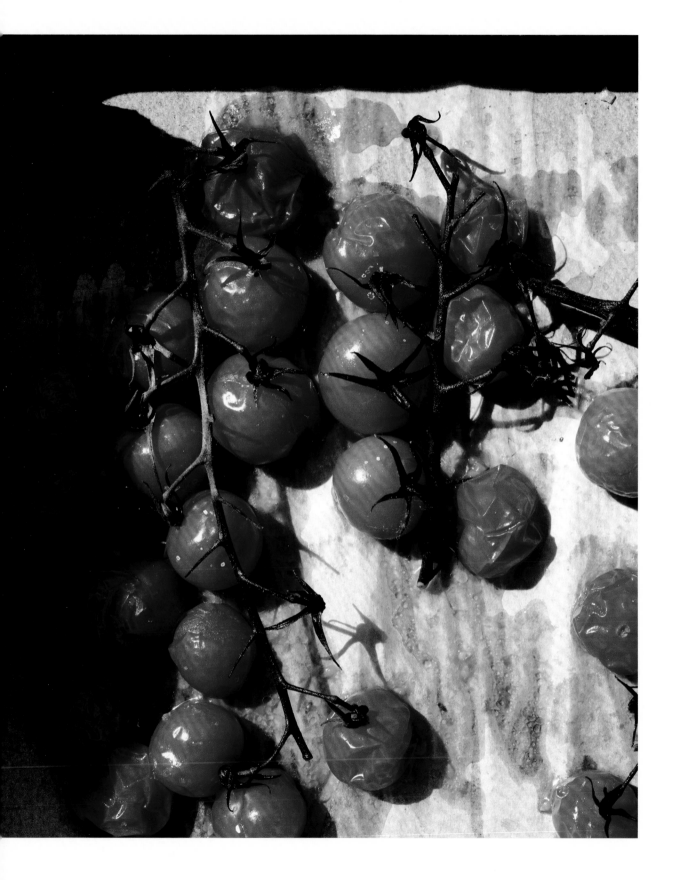

foods are prebiotics, so be sure to include in your weekly meals and snacks the specific prebiotic foods we mention above.

THE OTHER NUTRIENTS THAT SUPPORT YOUR MOOD

Polyphenols and Micronutrients

We know we need to eat more vegetables and fruits. One of the main reasons is that vegetables and fruits offer us polyphenols and micronutrients (i.e., vitamins and minerals).

Polyphenols

Polyphenols are what give plants their bright and beautiful colors, along with their scent and taste that act as natural defenses against insects or diseases as the plants are growing.[21] These protective mechanisms are powerful too when we eat them, helping our body defend against neurodegenerative disorders, cancer, heart disease, and possibly depression.[22] Polyphenols act like prebiotics in the gut—they help the good bacteria flourish and strengthen the gut lining.[23]

When you eat a wide variety of plants, especially colorful ones like vegetables and fruits, you know you're getting loads of polyphenols in your diet. A study found that when people increased their fruit and vegetable intake to eight portions a day, especially if they previously ate very few, they experienced more life satisfaction and their happiness levels increased substantially.[24]

Micronutrients

Micronutrients, also known as minerals and vitamins, are important nutrients that are found in small quantities in food yet play a massive role in overall health. Micronutrients are essential to the brain, nervous system, and mitochondria (think of these as the energizer bunnies that power each cell). They're found in all plants, not just fruits and veggies, and even in some dairy and meat products. There are *many* micronutrients that influence mood and mental health, and here we'll highlight a few key ones.

Magnesium

Magnesium is a mineral that helps calm the nervous system, regulates stress, relaxes muscles, aids in sleep, and helps ease anxiety and depression symptoms.[25] It does all this by regulating the body's circadian rhythm (which promotes deep sleep) and binding to GABA receptors (more on this neurotransmitter on page 24), creating a calming effect on the nervous system.[26] It's a nutrient that has a major influence on brain health; it's necessary for cognitive function and it will protect the brain as you age.[27] Magnesium has a lot of jobs to do—it's needed for over three hundred chemical reactions in your body![28] This may be why, when you are particularly stressed, your magnesium levels tend to become depleted as the body uses more of it.[29] Luckily, many of our recipes are filled with magnesium-rich foods to keep levels up.

Magnesium-rich foods: Pumpkin seeds, almonds, cashews, spinach and other leafy greens, avocados, black beans, dark chocolate, potatoes, brown rice, banana, salmon, and halibut.[30]

How much magnesium should you eat? We need between 310 and 420 mg of magnesium per day.

Sources of Magnesium

FOOD SOURCE	AMOUNT OF MAGNESIUM (MG)
¼ cup almonds	72
1 cup cooked black beans	120
1 cup cooked brown rice	83.9
1 oz dark (70–85%) chocolate	64
¼ cup pumpkin seeds	150
½ cup cooked spinach	78

B Vitamins

Similar to magnesium, B vitamins have a *lot* of different jobs in the body. These vitamins aid the body in maintaining a healthy nervous system, processing stress, producing energy, and building neurotransmitters (the ones responsible for feelings of happiness, pleasure, and calm).[31] While there are eight types of B vitamins, we focus here on three really important ones: B_6, B_9 (folate), and B_{12}.

Take vitamin B_6—it's essential in the production of neurotransmitters such as serotonin (the happiness neurotransmitter) and dopamine (the pleasure neuro-transmitter).[32] If B_6 levels are low, neurotransmitter production can be significantly impacted, and that's linked with a greater risk of depression.[33] Both B_9 (folate) and B_{12} are needed for proper nerve structure and function, and a deficiency of these two B vitamins is linked to depression.[34] Interestingly, B_{12} may even improve the effect of antidepressants when taken with them.[35] Just as with magnesium, stress tends to deplete some of the body's B vitamins, and deficiencies have been linked to greater risks of anxiety and depression.[36] Ensuring you eat B-vitamin-rich food is key—and lucky for you, our recipes are loaded with them.

B-vitamin-rich foods: beef liver, berries, brown rice, chicken, chickpeas, dark leafy greens, eggs, kefir, lentils, miso, peanuts, quinoa, salmon, sunflower seeds, sweet potato, tempeh, tuna, walnuts, and yogurt.

How much B-vitamin-rich food should you eat? You need varying amounts of each B vitamin (remember, there are eight of them), so mixing and matching B-vitamin-rich foods will help you cover your bases. For most adults, the recommended daily allowance (RDA)—the quantity deemed adequate to meet sufficient nutrient needs—for B_6, it's 1.3–1.5 mg; for B_9 (folate), it's 400 mcg (higher if pregnant); and for B_{12}, it's 2.4 mcg.

Sources of Vitamin B

FOOD SOURCE	AMOUNT OF B_6 (MG)
1 cup cooked chickpeas	1.1
1 cup cooked lentils	0.4
3 oz tuna	0.8

FOOD SOURCE	AMOUNT OF B_9 (FOLATE) (MCG)
4 spears cooked asparagus	88
1 cup cooked broccoli	163
1 cup cooked lentils	358

FOOD SOURCE	AMOUNT OF B_{12} (MCG)
3 oz ground beef	1.8
1 large egg	0.6 (mostly in the yolk)
3 oz salmon	2.7

Vitamin D

Vitamin D is known as the sunshine vitamin because it forms in the body when your skin is exposed to sunlight (but it's also found in some foods). If you live in a place that's dark and cold for many months out of the year (like we do!), your doctor has probably told you to take a vitamin D supplement. That's because vitamin D is used by every cell in the body, and it's difficult to get enough vitamin D through food alone (more on that later). Although vitamin D is mainly known for its role in building and maintaining healthy bones, it also has a big influence on the immune system, mood, and overall mental health. Many populations, from the elderly to pregnant women to teenagers, have been studied in order to explore the link between vitamin D and depression and anxiety.[37] The evidence is clear: vitamin D plays an essential role in mental well-being, and deficiencies may be linked to an increased risk of depression and anxiety.[38]

Vitamin D-rich foods: Vitamin D is found most abundantly in animal sources— butter, beef liver, egg yolks, salmon, sardines, trout, and tuna. It's also found in mushrooms, and oats. Non-dairy milk and dairy-free yogurt are often fortified with it. These latter, plant-based sources contain a form of vitamin D that doesn't raise levels as efficiently in the body, so it's better to get it from animal sources or a supplement.

How much vitamin D-rich food should you eat? The recommended daily allowance (RDA) for adults is 600 international units (IU), but you may need more depending on your health. It's best to talk with a healthcare practitioner to find out how much to supplement with.

Sources of Vitamin D

FOOD SOURCE	AMOUNT OF VITAMIN D (IU)
3 oz beef liver	42
1 large egg	44
3 oz rainbow trout	645

FOOD SOURCE	AMOUNT OF VITAMIN D (IU)
2 sardines	46
3 oz sockeye salmon	570
3 oz canned light tuna	40

Fat

The brain is composed of 60% fat, which makes fat a vital nutrient for brain function. Besides adipose tissue (otherwise known as body fat), it's the central nervous system, consisting of the brain and spinal cord, that has the highest concentration of fat in the entire body. And the central nervous system loves fat! More specifically, it loves PUFAS (polyunsaturated fatty acids), which you might know better as "omega-3" and "omega-6." These are essential fatty acids that our bodies can't make and must therefore get from food or supplements.

There are three main types of omega-3s:
- **DHA** (docosahexaenoic acid)
- **EPA** (eicosapentaenoic acid)
- **ALA** (alpha-linolenic acid)

DHA and EPA

DHA and EPA have been studied extensively for their influence on mood, mental health, memory, and cognitive function. They are needed for everyday brain function, help reduce inflammation in the brain, and are important components of brain cell membranes (membranes act like guardians controlling what enters and exits the cell).[39] They also play an important role in how messaging works between neurons. Plus they help lower cortisol (the main stress hormone).[40]

DHA and EPA are primarily found in fish and seafood (more on that on page 23). Eating more omega-3-rich foods has been shown to help with both depression and anxiety; consuming omega-3-rich fish, like salmon, is linked with a decreased risk of depression; and supplementing with a mixture of omega-3 and omega-6 may improve and even reduce anxious behavior.[41]

ALA

ALA is found in some plant foods, including chia seeds, flaxseeds, hemp seeds, and walnuts—that's why you'll often see the packaging of these foods claim that they're a good source of omega-3. These are extremely nutritious foods, and we highly recommend eating them. The body can convert ALA into DHA and EPA. This is a

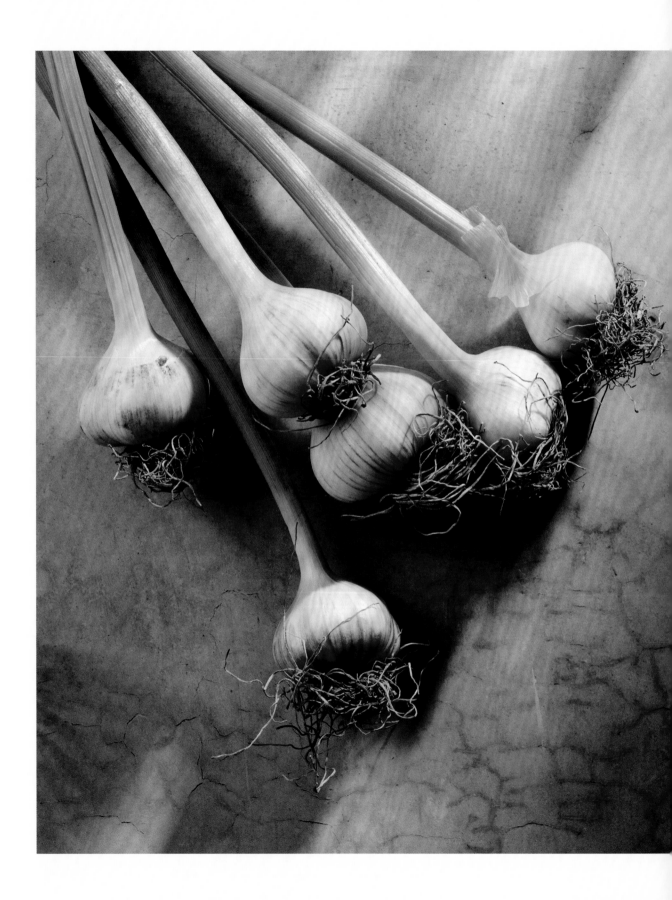

lengthy process that is not always easy or efficient for the body to do, so it's much more effective to consume DHA and EPA directly from food sources—that is, from the animal-based foods that contain them, like fish and seafood.

Omega-6: The Other Essential Fatty Acid

Omega-6 is also important for the nervous system and brain; it's abundant in foods commonly eaten in a Western diet, like grains, vegetable oils (such as sunflower, soy, and canola), and processed foods.[42] Most people are not deficient in omega-6 and in fact eat too much of it while eating too little omega-3—this has been linked with increased inflammation and chronic health issues.[43] When scientists have looked at people's blood levels, they can see that some people with anxiety and depression have a lower level of omega-3 and a higher ratio of omega-6.[44]

Omega-3-Rich Foods

- **Omnivore sources:** anchovies, cod, halibut, salmon, sardines, trout, tuna (albacore is much higher than skipjack).[45] If it's accessible, buy pasture-raised eggs and grass-fed beef, both of which are higher in omega-3 compared with animals raised on grains, which are higher in omega-6.
- **Plant-based sources:** chia seeds, flaxseeds, hemp seeds, and walnuts.

How much omega-3-rich food should you eat? It's recommended to consume 1.1–1.6 grams of ALA (the omega-3 found in plant foods) per day.[46] The Dietary Guidelines for Americans recommends eating 8 oz of fish or seafood per week to make sure you get DHA and EPA in your diet.[47] That looks like two 4-oz servings of salmon or other types of fish per week.

Sources of Omega-3

OMNIVORE FOOD SOURCES[48]	AMOUNT OF OMEGA-3 (G)
4 oz cod	0.19 (combined DHA and EPA)
4 oz salmon (farmed, Atlantic)	2.4 (combined DHA and EPA)
4 oz salmon (wild, Atlantic)	2.1 (combined DHA and EPA)
4 oz sardines	1.59 (combined DHA and EPA)
4 oz shrimp	0.32 (combined DHA and EPA)
4 oz canned light tuna	0.25 (combined DHA and EPA)

PLANT FOOD SOURCES[49]	AMOUNT OF OMEGA-3 (G)
2 Tbsp chia seeds	5.06 (ALA)
1 Tbsp whole flaxseeds	6.8 (ALA)
3 Tbsp hemp seeds	2.6 (ALA)
¾ cup walnuts	2.57 (ALA)

Protein

A robust gut microbiome will help build your neurotransmitters, since so many of them are produced there. However, there is another factor when it comes to supporting neurotransmitters: protein. As a quick reminder, neurotransmitters are chemical messengers that help your nerve cells talk to each other and deliver messages to feel calm, focused, or happy. Low levels of neurotransmitters can be a major contributor to mental illness and lowered mood states.[50]

You get amino acids from the protein consumed through your diet, and these help build neurotransmitters. Animal sources of protein will provide all the amino acids, whereas vegetarian sources of protein vary in the number of amino acids they contain. So, if you're vegetarian, you'll want to make sure you eat a variety of plant protein sources in order to consume all the different amino acids.

Why You Need Protein for Mood and Mental Wellness

Protein stabilizes blood sugar—this in turn impacts mood, anxiety, and depression (more on this on page 28). It is needed for the nervous system to function properly, to build healthy, balanced hormones and to make neurotransmitters.

The Neurotransmitters

Many types of neurotransmitters support mental wellness. The ones we focus on here are GABA (gamma-aminobutyric acid), serotonin, and dopamine. While many neurotransmitters are created in neurons (the cells of the nervous system, including the brain), a large number of them are made in the digestive tract by good microbes. There are specific strains of *Lactobacillus* and *Bifidobacterium* that actually make neurotransmitters—they do this by using nutrients from the food you eat: amino acids from protein, along with certain vitamins and minerals, including B_6 and zinc.[51]

GABA is often called the "calming neurotransmitter." Low levels of GABA are linked with anxiety, stress, and poor sleep.[52] Glutamine is the amino acid needed to make GABA.

Serotonin is known as the "happiness neurotransmitter." It helps you feel happy, relaxed, calm, and easygoing. The amino acid tryptophan eventually gets converted into serotonin, and a deficiency of tryptophan has been linked with depression.[53]

Dopamine helps you focus and feel motivated and energized, whether you're doing work, taking care of kids, or checking things off a to-do list. It's also known as the "pleasure chemical," or rather, the "anticipation of pleasure chemical"—it tells your brain to repeat behaviors that feel rewarding. Tyrosine is the amino acid needed to make dopamine.[54]

How much protein should you eat?
Most people may think they eat enough protein, but they usually don't. The recommended daily allowance (RDA) for

protein is 0.36 grams per pound of body weight per day. But most health professionals believe that number is too low and that it's actually closer to 0.50 to 1 gram per pound of body weight.

Sources of Protein

OMNIVORE FOOD SOURCES	AMOUNT OF PROTEIN (G)
4 oz beef	29
4 oz chicken breast	35
4 oz chicken thigh	27
4 oz cod	20
1 large egg	6
¼ cup feta cheese	5
1 cup plain Greek yogurt	16–19
4 oz lamb	30
4 oz salmon	23–30

PLANT FOOD SOURCES	AMOUNT OF PROTEIN (G)
2 Tbsp almonds	6.4
1 cup black beans	14
1 cup broccoli	2.5
2 Tbsp chia seeds	4.5
1 cup cooked chickpeas	10
3 Tbsp hemp seeds	9.5
1 cup cooked lentils	17
1 Tbsp peanut butter	2.4
2 Tbsp pumpkin seeds	9
½ cup quinoa	4
1 cup tempeh	34
¼ cup firm tofu	14
1 cup white beans	15

Sugar

Your brain loves sugar, that's because glucose is your brain's main fuel source (more on this in the next chapter, page 28). There's another reason too: when you consume sugar, it temporarily boosts your levels of serotonin and dopamine. This fills you with pleasure, reinforces to your brain how good that felt, and tells you to repeat the behavior (by eating another cookie, say, after you already had one or two or three). This reaction occurs with most sweet things, regardless of whether it's refined sugar or natural sugars from honey, coconut sugar, maple syrup, or dates.

Moderation Is Key

One reason you may want to be more moderate with your sugar intake is that what you eat feeds either good microbes or harmful microbes. Recent research shows that simple sugar (carbs that don't contain starch or fiber) profoundly impacts the gut microbes of mice. One study found that sugar increased the microbes that eat away at the gut mucus lining (not good!) and promoted the development of irritable bowel disease.[55]

Another study found that fructose and glucose (the building blocks of sugar) hinder some of our most important microbes from flourishing.[56] These may be rodent studies, but they still give us a window into our own health. Eating too much of any kind of sugar, whether it's refined sugar or honey, messes with blood sugar, and this may exacerbate feelings of stress and anxiety.

Should You Avoid Sugar Completely? (Hint: No)

In reality, we know it's tough to avoid sugar completely and, quite honestly, we wouldn't want to miss out on all the sweets and treats. The key, like with most things in life, is moderation. We want you to enjoy life and have dessert *and* still eat lots of whole, nourishing foods. The other key when it comes to enjoying sweets is to choose those made with natural sweeteners instead of processed ones. Unlike refined sugars, these healthier sweeteners still contain some nutrients, such as fiber, and some don't spike blood sugar nearly as high.

Natural Sweeteners to Enjoy

We recommend these natural sweeteners as alternatives to refined sugar:

- Coconut sugar or date sugar
- Sweet fruits like dates, bananas, and apples
- Small amounts of maple syrup and honey
- Stevia and monk fruit sweetener (these don't spike blood sugar at all)

THE BIG TAKEAWAYS

- Your gut microbes' favorite food is fiber, which is found only in plant foods. The microbes turn it into substances that help strengthen the communication between the gut and the brain, influencing your mood.
- Fermented foods, prebiotics, and resistant starches support these gut microbes.
- Polyphenols, found in colorful vegetables and fruits, and micronutrients including magnesium, B vitamins, and vitamin D, all uniquely support the nervous system and help protect against depression and anxiety.
- Fat, in the form of omega-3 and omega-6, supports brain health. Many people need to eat more omega-3.
- Protein helps build neurotransmitters—the chemical messengers that tell you to feel happy, alert, or calm.
- The brain loves sugar, but too much of it isn't a good thing. Stick to a moderate amount, to support a healthier gut microbiome and mood.

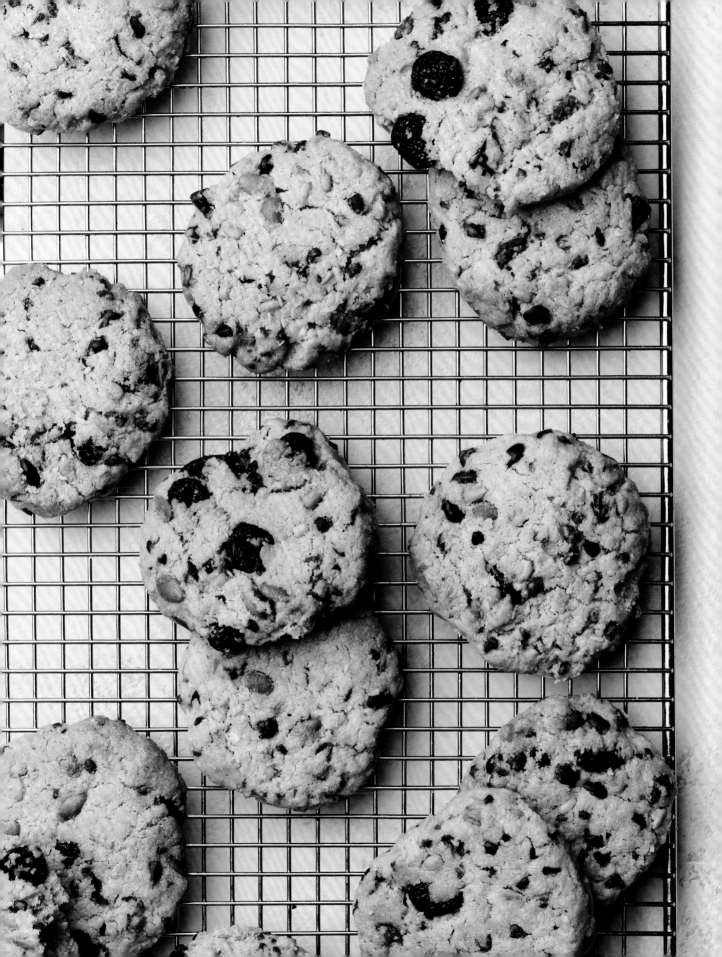

Balance Your Blood Sugar

Now, for one of our absolute favorite topics: blood sugar. You've most likely heard the phrase "Balance your blood sugar" (we've said similar phrases a bunch of times already in this book!); but what does that even mean? How do you do it? And why does it matter? We're about to explain, but first, we want to tell you about our client Samantha.

SAMANTHA'S STORY

Samantha is a mom to four kids. One of her kids has a disability, and she is constantly being pulled in seemingly a million different directions. She is in the middle of starting up her own business while also being a full-time parent and dealing with her own health challenges. She is capital B-U-S-Y.

When Samantha would get particularly stressed, which happened often, she would grab whatever carby thing was in sight—cold hash browns left on her kid's plate from breakfast or leftover Halloween candy, for example. Often, she'd eat a few extra pieces of pizza for dinner, even though she already felt stuffed. And then something interesting would happen. Every time she ate foods that skyrocketed her blood sugar (like the ones mentioned above), she would become very, very anxious. She would have heart

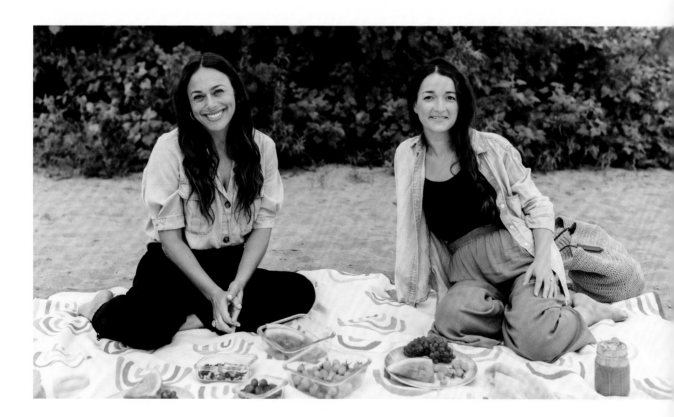

palpitations, her head would start pounding, fatigue would set in, and she would become even more stressed. And although she felt horrible, she just figured it was because she was capital B-U-S-Y.

When we started working together and looking closely at her diet, we connected the dots: whenever she ate foods that spiked her blood sugar, her mood, anxiety, and cravings became much worse. It took time, but we worked on her diet, putting the focus on keeping her blood sugar stable. And guess what? Her anxiety started to lessen. She said it felt like a fog was lifting. She emailed us about this breakthrough, saying, "I can't believe it—my anxiety, headaches, and intense fatigue are disappearing! It finally hit me that food definitely impacts how I feel in a huge way. I am actually shocked!"

We know, we know, this sounds so simplistic—balance your blood sugar and *poof*—anxiety begone! Of course, it's not going to be the same for everyone—blood sugar balance isn't always the magical key that alleviates anxiety, but it sure can help, *a lot*. It can also help keep mood steady, ease depressive feelings, maintain or enhance cognitive function and memory, prevent heart palpitations, lessen irritability, and reduce cravings.[57]

WAIT, WHAT *IS* BLOOD SUGAR?

"Balance your blood sugar" is a phrase that is often thrown around, but you might not intrinsically understand what this entails. Before we explain how to balance blood sugar, let's first revisit tenth-grade biology.

You eat something that has carbohydrates in it. Regardless of whether it's something that's high in sugar or refined carbs (like doughnuts, muffins, or spaghetti), or something that's a complex carb (like sweet potatoes, chickpeas, or apples)—the food is broken down into molecules, including glucose (sugar), by your digestive system. Glucose is the main fuel source for your body—your brain not only *loves* it, it *needs* it to survive. And when glucose converts into energy, this isn't just energy for us to feel alert, awake, and energized, it's energy that our body uses for *everything*—from thinking to blinking to the heart beating.

As soon as the glucose is in your blood, your pancreas senses this and releases a hormone called insulin. (If you have type 1 diabetes, your body does not make insulin and so you have to inject it into your body.) Insulin's job is to get glucose into your cells so that it can be used for energy. Insulin also tells glucose exactly where to go and if it needs to be stored.

But what happens when you eat something with lots of simple carbs and very little fiber (like a sugar cookie or a croissant), known as a high glycemic index food? Since there are so few nutrients and fiber in it, it breaks down into glucose quickly, and now you have *lots* of glucose in your blood. The pancreas releases insulin to tell glucose where to go ASAP. The insulin then puts some of the glucose into the cells to be used immediately. But there is too much glucose—the body can't just keep the extra in the blood; that's dangerous, so it needs to find somewhere to dump it. So some gets stored in the liver and in the muscles (which is short-term storage with limited capacity), and if there's still excess glucose, the body converts it into fat, for which there is a ton of storage space.

WHAT'S THE PROBLEM WITH UNSTABLE BLOOD SUGAR?

Most of us ride the blood sugar or glucose roller coaster all day long. Imagine that for breakfast you eat a piece of toast with some almond butter, banana slices, and honey drizzled on top. This may seem like a filling breakfast—it's got some fiber and some fat. But for most people, it converts into glucose pretty quickly—most likely because there isn't enough protein in this meal (see more about that on page 24). This spikes blood sugar (glucose) high, and then crashes it down soon after.

Once it crashes, the cravings come on, usually for something carby to help get your blood sugar back up. You reach for a snack, but because your blood sugar is low and you may be feeling a bit *hangry*, you choose something that's fairly sugary—after all, it's easier and more appetizing to grab a few crackers or a muffin than it is to munch on veggies. Your brain knows these types of foods will raise your blood sugar quickly and offer immediate energy for the body, so it craves them. But you just got back on the roller coaster. Your blood sugar spikes, and then crashes, and this continues throughout the day, informing most, if not all, of your food choices until you go to bed. Blood sugar can also impact quality of sleep, and without good sleep, say hello to a cranky, tired, irritable you the next day.

What's also happening is that with every spike and crash, you may experience irritability, tingling extremities, heart palpitations, lack of focus, extreme fatigue, fogginess, headache, heaviness over your eyes, lethargy, feelings of anxiousness, and sometimes deep sadness.[58] It hits each person differently, but these are common side effects of the roller coaster. For some, these side effects may be much more pronounced than for others.

RIDING THE ROLLER COASTER

This pattern of continuous blood sugar ups and downs may over time lead to insulin resistance, which is when your cells no longer respond to insulin quickly, leaving your blood sugar elevated for longer periods. Unfortunately, this is incredibly common—about one out of every three American adults age 18 and older experience this—and it's a major risk factor for type 2 diabetes, among many other health conditions.[59] Insulin resistance is also linked with mood disorders; a group of Stanford scientists found that insulin resistance doubles the risk of depression in adults.[60]

When scientists removed insulin receptors from the brains of mice (glucose gets into cells through these receptors), it triggered depressive and anxiety-like behaviors.[61] Although the test subjects were mice, the research gives us insight into the human body and its reaction. The brain loves sugar (which you'll recall from page 25), and if sugar (glucose) does not properly get into brain cells because of insulin resistance, this may lead to cognitive decline and memory issues.[62]

IS IT STRESS OR IS IT BLOOD SUGAR IMBALANCE?

Many clients we work with don't realize that feeling tired, irritable, sad, or anxious could be connected to their blood sugar. Rather, they usually attribute it to work stress, parenting, or getting older—or think it's just their normal baseline. A great way to check in with your body is to see how your meals and snacks are affecting your blood sugar 1–2 hours after you eat. Ask yourself: "How am I feeling after this meal?" Are you experiencing cravings for carby foods, sweets, or coffee 1–2 hours after eating? Are you tired, hungry again, or even feeling starving? If you're nodding your head to say "That's me," it's time to balance your blood sugar. For those of you who don't experience that, it could be that you've been on the blood sugar roller coaster for so long, you're no longer even aware that you're on the ride. So, even if you're not nodding your head, you most likely could still benefit from eating foods that help balance blood sugar.

BALANCING BLOOD SUGAR

Balancing or steadying your blood sugar (glucose) means that you won't be experiencing major spikes and crashes throughout the day. The key is to choose nourishing sources of carbohydrates: root vegetables (like sweet potatoes, parsnips, beets), beans and other legumes, and whole grains (like quinoa and steel-cut oats). Eat these carbohydrates in combination with protein (like chicken, fish, eggs, lentils, or hemp seeds), fiber (like legumes, vegetables and fruits), and fat (like nuts, seeds, extra virgin olive oil, avocado, or coconut). This combination slows the speed at which the carbs break down into glucose and in turn spike insulin, because protein, fat, and fiber are structurally more complex than simple or starchy carbs and take longer for your body to break down. This will ensure your brain is well fueled, which means better focus and productivity, more steady energy, and balanced moods. And luckily, the recipes in this cookbook were specifically developed with this in mind and will help you achieve this balance.

HOW TO EAT SWEETS WITHOUT SPIKING YOUR BLOOD SUGAR

You don't need to cut out carbs, or say goodbye to sweets either. When it comes to desserts and treats, we still eat them, and there are two ways to make sweets more supportive of blood sugar balance. First, by including protein, fiber, and fat in your desserts; we'll show you how to do this in the desserts chapter (page 189). Second, if you eat a balanced meal of protein, fat, and fiber first, and then you eat a sugary dessert after, it won't spike your blood sugar as high as it otherwise would. Meaning you're not as likely to experience a big blood sugar spike and crash.

THE PLATE CHECK

One method of eating that we share with our clients is called the plate check. Three things need to be present on the plate when you eat. There can be foods outside of these categories, of course, but these three items must be present:

- **Protein:** About 20–40 grams per meal (depending on activity level), from foods such as beef, chicken, eggs, fish, legumes, tempeh and tofu.
- **Fat:** 1–3 tablespoons of foods such as avocado, coconut, extra virgin olive oil, nuts, olives, seeds and tahini.
- **Colorful fruits and vegetables:** When you eat a variety of veggies, your body gets a variety of nutrients, as well as fiber (and, as we know, fiber feeds those good gut bugs!). Aim for at least 2 cups of raw vegetables if you're having a salad, and at least 1 cup of cooked vegetables if you're having a cooked side. Feel free to fill up any extra space on your plate with more vegetables!

THE BIG TAKEAWAYS

- Riding the blood sugar roller coaster all day may lead to anxiety, stress, lowered mood, and eventually insulin resistance.
- Insulin resistance has been linked with cognitive decline, depression, and anxiety.
- Balanced blood sugar allows you to feel satiated for longer, and helps create steady energy and a stable mood.
- Balancing blood sugar is not about cutting out sugar completely; rather, it's about eating it with protein, fiber, and fat to lessen the glucose spike and maintain a steady mood.

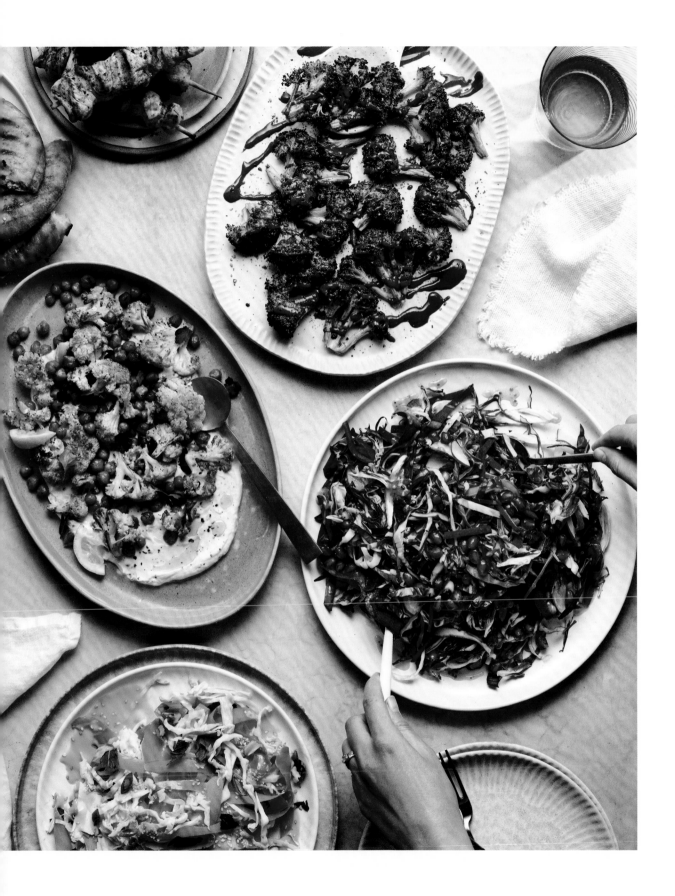

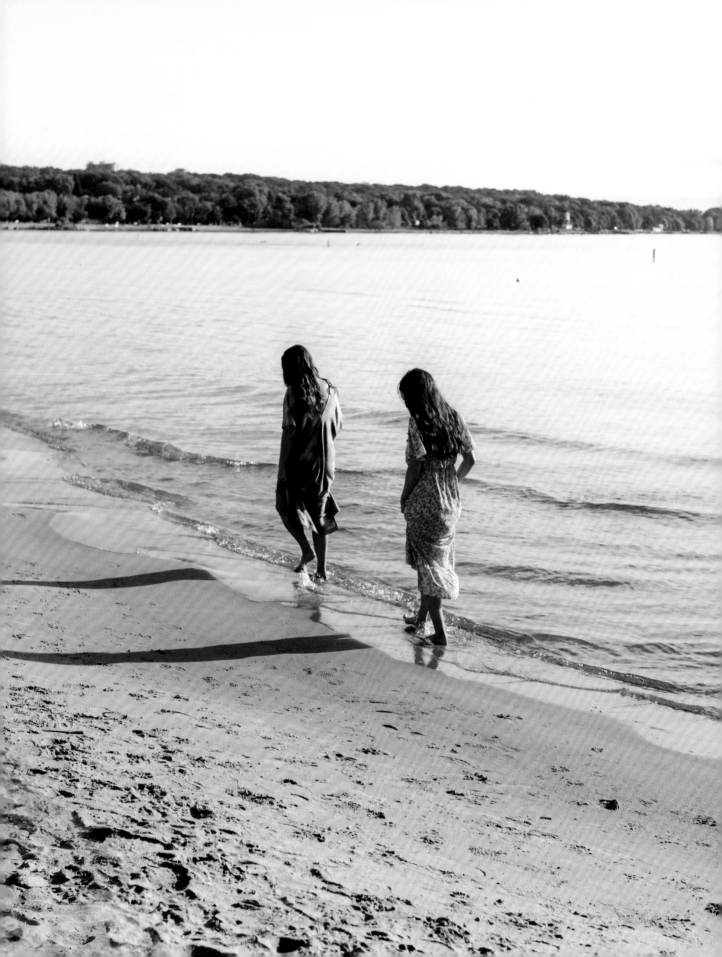

Putting It All into Practice

In the previous chapters, we gave you *a lot* of information on how what you eat greatly impacts how you feel. Now you might be wondering, *How do I implement all this information in my daily life?* You might be thinking, *I now need to eat way more fiber, eat protein at all my meals, include more colorful vegetables and fermented foods, figure out how to balance my blood sugar, and I have to do this every day?!*

Now that we have the knowledge, we need to actually put it into practice. Many of us know what to do; the hard part is doing what we know. *If I know this is good for me, why can't I seem to do it?* Or alternatively, *If I know this isn't good for me, why do I do it?* Sound familiar? We may have a surge of willpower or motivation, but then, for most of us, that fizzles out pretty quickly, because life happens and derails us.

The way to implement what you know in your daily life is . . . kind of boring. We wish there were a more pizzazz-filled kind of way, but there's not. When it comes to eating better to support your mental health, there's the action part—the actual eating. And then there's the mental part—building a healthy food mindset (which we'll get to soon).

THE ACTION PART

The action part is about building habits like eating consistently throughout the day, making intentional choices to add veggies, protein, and/or fiber to a meal, ensuring there are groceries in the fridge, and having some plan in mind about what to cook and eat. Ask yourself these questions, to start building this habit:

- Am I skipping meals—lunch, for instance?
- Do I spend the day grazing on snacks instead of eating whole meals?
- Am I drinking enough water (8 to 12 cups of water per day)?
- Is protein a part of every single one of my meals?
- How much protein am I actually eating?
- Am I eating a variety of colorful plants throughout the week?
- Do I have time to prep and cook food? If not, where can I find a meal delivery service, or pick up prepared foods that support my health?
- Am I eating too many simple carbs (such as cookies, pasta, or chips), which are giving my body more energy than it needs or demands?
- Do I crave the same thing at the same time every single day (like coffee or chocolate at 3 p.m.)?
- Am I even hungry before I eat, or am I just bored—or tired, anxious, excited, or procrastinating?
- Am I full, satisfied, stuffed, or bloated after I eat?
- Do I fall into a now-I-must-unbutton-my-pants food coma after eating?
- How do I feel 1–2 hours after I eat?

These may seem like a lot of questions, and if you're someone who experiences over-whelm, you may be thinking, *Ah, I don't know! This is a lot!* That's okay. Breathe, dear reader! This isn't the shame game here. No one is judging you because you forgot to drink water today or you've been subsisting on handfuls of nuts instead of whole meals. But this is an amazing starting place for you to understand where you're at right now.

For healthy eating habits, here are answers to some of the questions above:

- I eat 2–3 main meals throughout the day and nourishing snacks (rather than grazing every 1–2 hours).
- My meals are filled with 20–40 grams of protein, fiber-rich colorful veggies and/or fruit, and some good fat.
- I wait 2½–3½ hours between meals to allow for digestion, but listen to my body and eat sooner if I need to.
- I eat a protein-rich snack or a mini-meal before 3 p.m. if I'm prone to the afternoon crash and know it's coming.
- I drink 8 to 12 cups of water per day.
- I chew my food, slow down, and feel satisfied after eating, rather than bloated or stuffed.

Build the Habits

As with many things in life, repetition and consistency are key. If you're trying to build more muscle, you must repeat exercises that stimulate your muscles—and do it often. If you're trying to learn how to play guitar or learn a new language, you must practice a lot.

Putting all this knowledge into place takes practice and, luckily, because you eat several times a day every single day, you have plenty of time to practice this and work it out. As James Clear, the author of *Atomic Habits*, says, "It is so easy to dismiss the value of making slightly better decisions on a daily basis. Sticking with the funda-mentals is not impressive. Falling in love with boredom is not sexy. Getting one percent better isn't going to make headlines."[63] But small daily changes, like drinking more water, eating more protein, and including more colorful plants on your plate, create enormous positive impacts for your body and mind over time.

THE MINDSET PART

Now comes the food mindset part (and by the way, this is a much bigger conversation than this short section covers). For some people, this may require deeper work with a professional. But we'll give you a starting point.

We first realized how necessary this food mindset part is when clients of ours came to us berating and bullying themselves. They would tell us how mad, disappointed, frustrated, and disgusted they were with themselves after they ate foods they deemed as "junk" or "bad," or if they felt they'd fallen "off the wagon" or got "off track." Or if they'd not eaten a vegetable that day or drunk more than a few sips of water. Or they'd compare their body with someone else's. So many of us are incredibly hard on ourselves. Our inner dialogue can be harsh—we would never dream of saying the things we say to ourselves to a friend, or a child, or even a complete stranger.

For years, we've worked on our own food mindset, rewriting our narrative around diets, health, and what healthy bodies "should" look like. Eventually, we created a method for ourselves and our clients for building a healthier relationship with food. Let's look at this step-by-step method now.

Step One: Be Your Own Detective

The first step is uncovering what meanings, stories, and beliefs you may have unconsciously created and repeated over and over again about eating certain foods, food labels (like "good," "bad," "clean," "junk"), portions, mealtimes, family gatherings, and bodies.

Here are examples from our clients:
- Family members would make inappropriate and unwelcome comments about their portion sizes and body. Now they're incredibly self-conscious about how much they eat and what they look like.
- Mealtime was filled with anxiety and stress because they were forced to finish everything on their plate, even when they were extremely full. Now they have a hard time paying attention to their hunger cues and tend to overeat at every meal.
- They weren't allowed any "junk food" in the house when growing up. Now they don't know how to have treats in the house without binging on them.
- They were taught that food is simply a tool to shrink themselves rather than to nourish, fuel, and energize themselves, and enhance their health. Now they feel confused about what's "healthy" and jump from one fad diet to another.

Maybe you see yourself in these stories or maybe you don't. Either way, it's a good time to get curious and explore your thoughts, stories, patterns, judgments, phrases, habits, and assumptions you have about food that may be stuck on auto-play in your mind.

Step Two: Question If It's True

Years ago, we heard a mother at a preschool say to her child, "Just because someone said it, doesn't make it true." This has stuck with us ever since. It's true of our thoughts as well: just because you think it, doesn't make it true.

If you just binged on something, overate or underate at a meal, ate too many sweets, or looked in the mirror and felt disappointed and then began judging, shaming, or berating yourself, this is the perfect time to question what you're thinking: Is it true? Usually, the deeper reason people shame themselves is that they're trying to use it as a motivation so that they don't repeat the behavior. But when has bullying yourself ever really worked as motivation in the long term? Probably never. And remember, just because you think it, doesn't make it true!

Step Three: Stop, Drop, and Feel Your Feelings

It's time to stop, drop, breathe, and feel. One of our teachers once said that the breath digests feelings just like the digestive system digests food. Breathing helps you pause and gives you time and space to feel the physical sensation of your feelings and tell your nervous system you're safe. Close your eyes and take a few deep breaths, notice what sensations and feelings you have going on inside, or if any old memories or thoughts are coming up. What does it physically feel like in your body? Tight? Hot? Tense? Loose? Tingly? Breathe into these sensations and just feel them fully, without trying to get rid of them or judging them.

Then ask yourself, "What do I *need* right now?"

Maybe it's:
- Something physical like going for a walk, stretching, dancing, shaking, or doing jumping jacks.
- Quieting down with deep breathing, doing a two-minute meditation, or firmly placing your hand on your chest.
- Calling a friend, or journaling, or saying all the things you're thinking out loud.
- A good cry or yell to release whatever is upsetting you.
- Listening to music or watching a hilarious show.

Once you've done something to feel the feelings, they usually have less of a hold on you. You might find that bringing awareness to what's happening emotionally allows you to change these patterns.

Step Four: Celebrate Your Small Wins

Most people are really hard on themselves and blind to all of the things they are *already* doing well. It's as if they have hawk eyes that can spot their flaws, mistakes, and setbacks from miles away yet they can't see all the small daily wins that are right in front of them. Acknowledging and celebrating these positives is a wonderful way to build confidence, boost mood, and flood the body with feel-good neurotransmitters. Regularly praising yourself boosts motivation to repeat the activities again and primes your brain to look for success.

Here's what we consider small wins:
- You drank water today.
- You ate a meal that included colorful vegetables.
- You went for a walk or moved your body in some way.
- You ate chocolate and loved every bite.

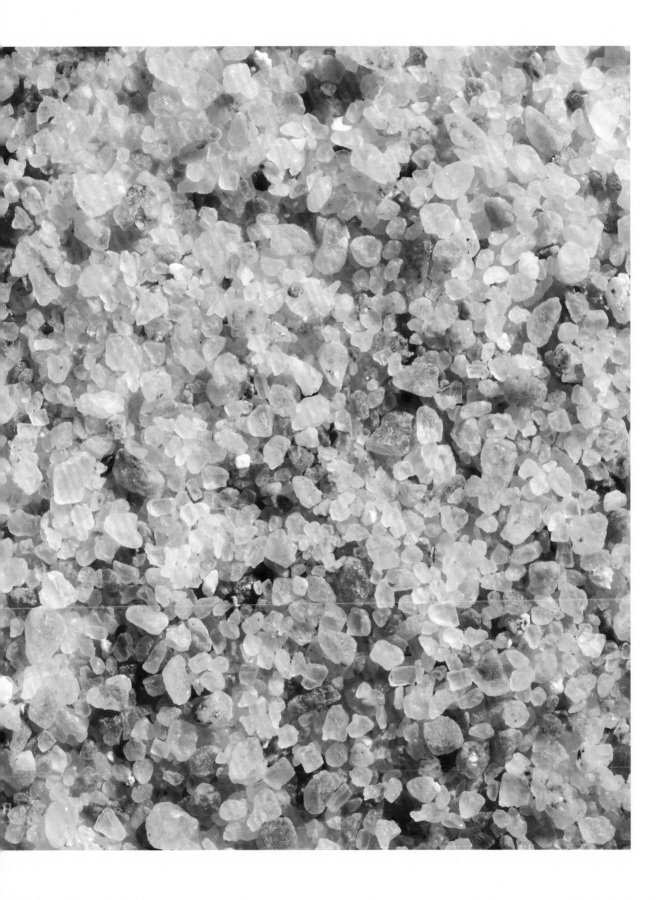

- You didn't skip any meals that day.
- You stopped eating when you felt full.
- You fully enjoyed a meal out with friends.

Your days are filled to the brim with wins, and celebrating them is a far greater motivator than anything else. If you're feeling particularly low, see if you can recall a few small wins, or make that a daily practice by reflecting at the end of each day on five things you did well that day.

This mindset part is just as important as the action part. The thoughts you think and the words you say (whether internally or out loud) about what you eat, how you eat, how you cook, how you look, and even how you meal plan and grocery shop dictates how you behave and act. So be kind to yourself, celebrate your wins, and, now, let's cook some good food!

HOW TO USE THIS BOOK

In the first part of *Good Food, Good Mood* we've given you *a lot* of information on the science behind the foods you eat, and now we put all that research into our recipes. *Good Food, Good Mood*'s recipes are divided into chapters on breakfasts, snacks, mains, sides, desserts, and drinks. The meals, snacks, drinks, and even desserts are designed to support blood sugar balance, include a variety of colorful plants and fermented foods to feed good bacteria in the gut, and boast lots of protein to produce neurotransmitters and keep you feeling fuller for longer. If you're anything like us, you love to cook but you don't always have hours to spend in the kitchen. We've designed most of these recipes to be fairly simple—they have short ingredient lists and can be prepared quickly.

In the **Breakfasts chapter**, the recipes focus on fiber and protein—making these nutrients a part of your first meal will set the tone for the rest of your day. Together, they regulate your appetite so it's easier to make healthier food choices throughout the day. They help you feel steady and energized, and the protein builds neurotransmitters, making you feel alert and focused. We know that mornings can feel rushed, so some of the recipes take only minutes to prepare; others can be made ahead of time, stored in the freezer or fridge, and heated up quickly when you're ready to eat.

The **Snacks chapter** includes recipes for dips, crackers, and breads. It may seem daunting to make these recipes from scratch—why wouldn't you just buy them at the store? We promise that they're much faster and easier than you think, and far more tasty and nutritious.

The recipes in the **Mains chapter** are organized by their protein source: fish, plants, or meat. We tend to eat the heartiest meals with the most protein and veggies during dinner or lunch, so that's the focus of our mains. The dishes are delicious, most are brimming with plants (to help you rack up your fiber points!) and, of course, protein to help produce feel-good neurotransmitters and avoid major mood dips by keeping blood sugar stable. Many of the recipes are quick to make, and some use just one pot or pan for extra ease and easy cleanup. Many of the mains have side dishes built into the recipes, but for those that don't, pair them with a recipe from the **Sides chapter**. To save time, eat dinner leftovers for lunch the next day.

The point of the **Sides chapter** is to help you eat more plants—and we believe *they must be delicious*. From page 14, you know that eating a variety of plants (as in over 30 a week), fermented foods, and polyphenols help support a diverse and healthy microbiome. These healthy gut bugs go on to influence behavior and mood. The recipes in this chapter—ranging from raw, flavorful slaws and salads to warming, cooked vegetables and soups—will help you feel good from the inside out. Many of the sides pair well with the mains—and we've provided suggestions in the recipes—but mix-and-match what appeals to you!

The recipes in the **Desserts chapter** are meant to be yummy without making you feel crummy after eating them. We incorporate healthy fats and protein from almonds, tahini, and yogurt; fiber from beans, oats, fruit; and sweeteners from dates, bananas, and coconut sugar to make delicious desserts that are better for your blood sugar. Whether you feel like preparing cookies, breads, brownies, tarts, or gummies, we've got the recipe for you.

The **Drinks chapter** offers you recipes for something warm and cozy, or cool and refreshing, as well as for filling smoothies in case you want to enjoy a more substantial beverage with breakfast or as a snack. You'll find colorful fruits and vegetables included in these drinks, along with fermented foods and nourishing fats, to make your drinks nutrient-dense and mood-supporting.

INGREDIENTS WE LIKE TO USE

Here's a roundup of the staple items we tend to keep in our kitchens and use often in the recipes in this book.

Oils

We like to use extra virgin olive oil, unrefined coconut oil, and butter in most of our cooking. We use extra virgin olive oil for dressings and sauces, but it also works well for sautéing and roasting. We love using unrefined coconut oil and butter in baking and dessert recipes. We also use unrefined coconut oil for cooking vegetables and making soups, if the coconut flavor works well. Occasionally, we use toasted sesame oil to add extra flavor to dressings.

Vinegars and Seasonings

We often use balsamic vinegar and rice vinegar in our recipes and occasionally apple cider vinegar, red wine vinegar, and white wine vinegar. We always have tamari (you could use coconut aminos, if you can't eat soy), a good-quality mayonnaise, and Dijon or grainy mustard on hand in our kitchens.

Flours and Grains

You'll find that we most often use gluten-free flours, such as almond flour, when cooking for clients, since most of them are sensitive to gluten. Almond flour is rich in healthy fats and has some protein, which we love to include in dishes to stabilize blood sugar. We also use oat flour frequently, since it's affordable and readily available (certified gluten-free oat flour is available too). You'll also find buckwheat flour, tapioca starch (or arrowroot starch), and chickpea flour (sometimes labeled as "garbanzo bean flour") used in some of our recipes, because it's relatively high in protein and fiber. On occasion, we use whole grain flours like rye and spelt. As for oats, we tend to use rolled and steel-cut in our breakfast recipes. We use short grain brown rice, but you can always swap in long grain brown rice, if that's what you have. And lastly, we use quinoa occasionally.

Dairy and Eggs

- **Milk:** Our recipes call for "milk of choice." We prefer plant-based milks like coconut milk, almond milk, and macadamia nut milk, but you should choose based on your preference. Make sure to get unsweetened varieties of plant-based milks to avoid any added sugar.
- **Yogurt:** If your diet is dairy-free, you can use a coconut-based yogurt in our recipes, but make sure it's unsweetened. For dairy yogurt, we like Greek yogurt, since it's higher in protein than regular yogurt. We also love sheep and goat milk yogurt—if you can find that, give it a try!
- **Eggs:** We like to use organic, pasture-raised eggs, but we know those can be expensive, so free-range eggs are another good option that's more affordable. Large-sized eggs work well in our recipes.

Fish and Seafood

We try to buy wild-caught or sustainably farmed fish and seafood. These types of fish can be a little bit more expensive, but they are nutrient-dense and ensure the fish are coming from healthy environments that are better for humans and the sustainability of our oceans.

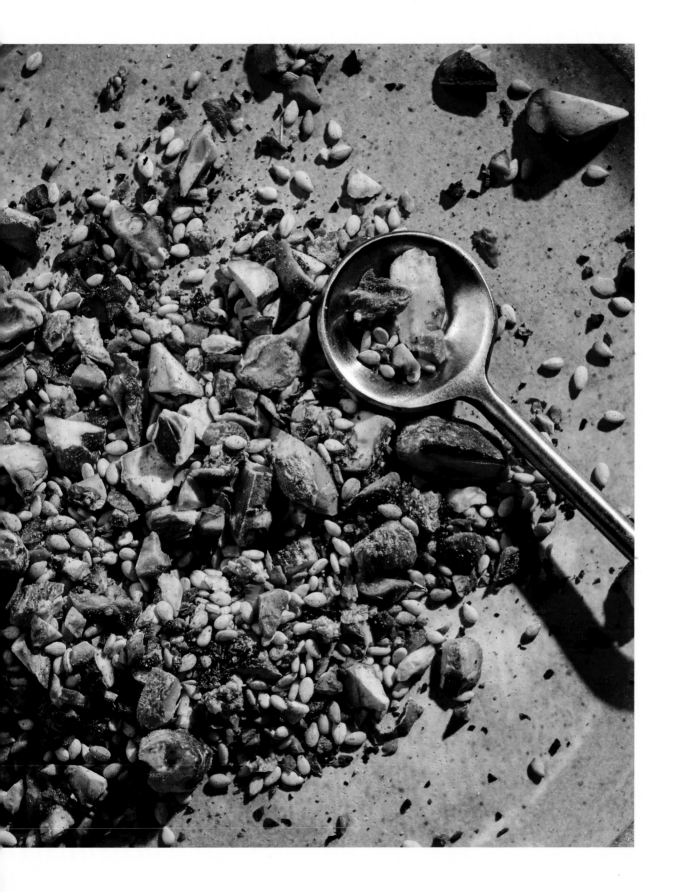

Meat and Poultry

When possible, we buy meat and poultry from local farms. Even if they aren't certified organic, many local farms raise their animals in the same way organic farms do—with access to the outdoors, and pasture-raised and grass-fed, without antibiotics and hormones. If that's not available where you are, look for free-range chicken and meat that's free of antibiotics and hormones.

Legumes

You'll find a variety of legumes in our recipes, including chickpeas, black beans, white beans, kidney beans, and lentils, as well as tempeh (made from fermented soybeans). We usually keep cans of beans in our pantries to make meal prep quick and easy. We buy red, green, French, and beluga lentils in bulk.

Nuts and Seeds

We keep a variety of nuts and seeds in stock at home, especially almonds, cashews, walnuts, chia seeds, flaxseeds, hemp seeds, and pumpkin seeds. Feel free to use any other nuts and seeds that you love in our recipes—or just have them around for snacking on. We also love tahini and always have it around, as well as nut butter, such as almond butter or peanut butter.

Fermented Foods

If you have the time to make your own ferments, such as sauerkraut, from scratch, that's amazing! We are huge fans of homemade fermented foods such as sauerkraut, lacto-fermented pickles, sourdough, and yogurt. We usually don't have the time to make these foods from scratch, so we buy our fermented foods—including sauerkraut, lacto-fermented pickles, kimchi, and miso—at the grocery store; these particular ferments should be located in the refrigerator section to preserve their probiotics.

Sweeteners

We use pure maple syrup, coconut sugar, honey, dates, and fruits like berries, apples, and bananas to sweeten our recipes.

RECIPE MOOD AND NUTRIENT BENEFITS

On each recipe page, you'll find a list of mood and nutrient benefits for that recipe.

Mood Benefits

+ **Calm:** Feel peaceful, tranquil, and less stressed.
+ **Energize:** Feel a boost (without relying on caffeine!).
+ **Focus:** Feel attentive, clear, and less overwhelmed.
+ **Sleep:** Feel relaxed and ready for deep, restorative rest.
+ **Uplift:** Feel positive, joyful, and cheery.

Nutrient Benefits

+ **Blood Sugar Balancer:** Will keep blood sugar stable and steady with a combination of protein, fat, and/or fiber.
+ **Colorful:** Includes ingredients that are colorful, micronutrient-rich plants and polyphenols.
+ **Fermented:** Includes fermented, probiotic-rich foods.
+ **Fiber-Rich:** Includes ingredients loaded in fiber to support blood sugar balance and beneficial gut bacteria.
+ **Healthy Fats:** Includes omega-3s and/or nutritious fats to support the brain and nervous system.
+ **Prebiotic:** Good source of plant fibers that help beneficial bacteria flourish in the gut.
+ **Protein-Powered:** Amino acid–rich foods that are needed for neurotransmitters and blood sugar balance.

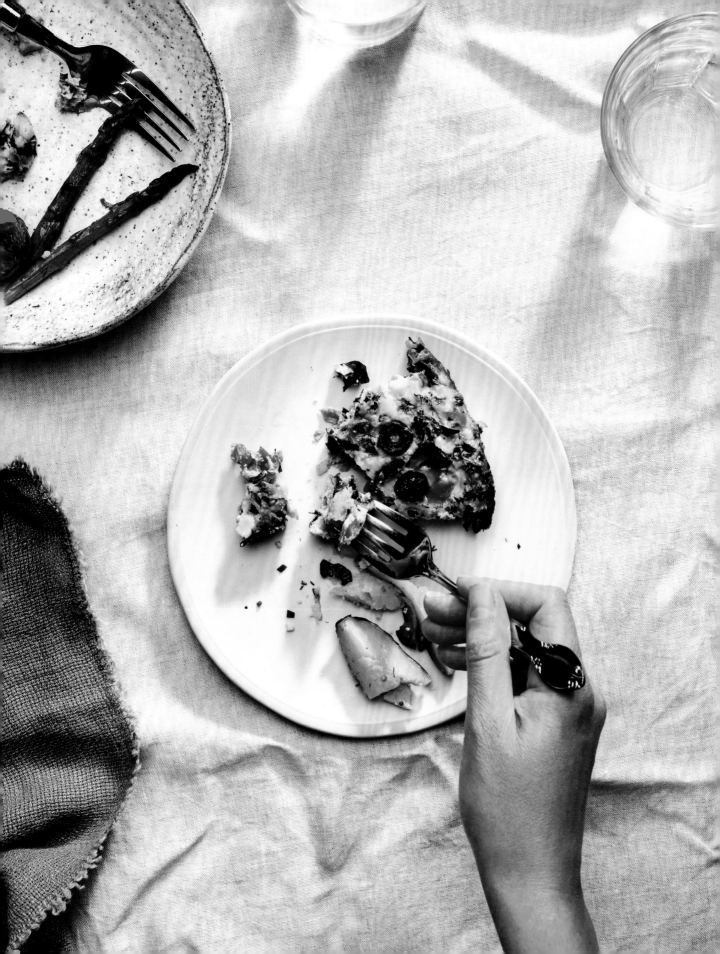

breakfasts

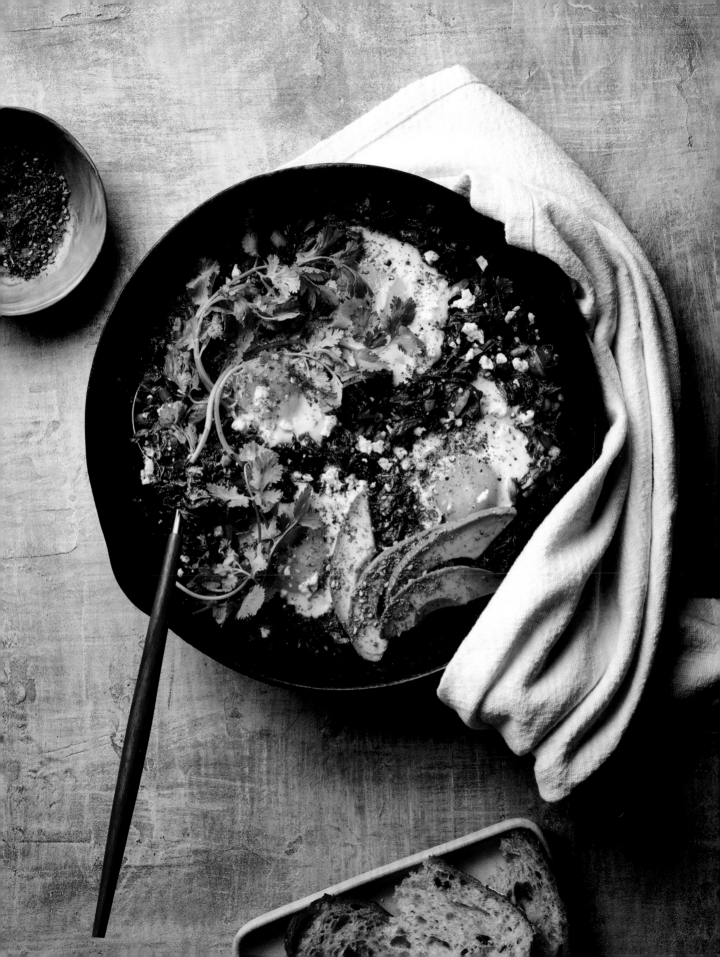

Green Shakshuka

1 Tbsp extra virgin olive oil

1 small yellow onion, diced

2 garlic cloves, sliced

1 tsp ground cumin

6 cups chopped green veggies of choice (we like a combo of kale, Swiss chard, and zucchini)

½ tsp sea salt

A few cracks of pepper

4 eggs (you can use up to 8 eggs, if you like)

TOPPINGS (CHOOSE THE ONES YOU LOVE THE MOST)

Fresh herbs (cilantro, flat-leaf parsley, mint, dill, basil)

½–1 avocado, peeled, pitted, and sliced

¼ cup crumbled feta

A few dollops of harissa paste

A few spoonfuls of dairy or dairy-free yogurt

Broken crusty sourdough bread

A few dashes of hot sauce

A pinch of za'atar

⊕ **ENERGIZE, FOCUS, UPLIFT**

PREP TIME: 5 MINUTES   **COOK TIME:** 20 MINUTES   **SERVES:** 2–4

If you've enjoyed shakshuka before, you most likely had the version in which eggs are slowly poached in a delicious, Middle Eastern spiced tomato sauce. This recipe is a bit different, and it's a favorite of ours and many of our clients. It's an easy way to get a lot of greens into your body, and it's quite forgiving—you can use whatever greens you love or have on hand. Protein-rich eggs combined with fibrous green veggies energize the mind and body and help keep your mood steady for hours. What makes this recipe sing are the toppings, so be sure to choose at least one.

1 Place a large, wide skillet over medium-high heat, add the oil, and swirl it around to coat the bottom. Toss in the onion and sauté until translucent, about 3–5 minutes.

2 Add the garlic, sauté for another minute until fragrant. Sprinkle in the cumin and stir. Place the greens in the pan. If there are too many to fit, work in batches, adding a few handfuls at a time. Allow the greens to wilt before adding the next batch.

3 Season with salt and pepper and allow the greens to wilt completely and cook down, about 5–7 minutes.

4 Make little wells in the greens and crack in the eggs. We like to use 4 eggs, but you can add up to 8 if your pan is big enough. After a minute, cover the pan for about 5 minutes so the eggs cook. If you don't have a lid big enough, use a smaller lid that partially covers the pan, just as long as the eggs are covered. Cook the eggs for longer, if that's your preference. If you're a fan of runny yolks, watch the eggs closely so they don't overcook.

5 Serve the shakshuka with your toppings of choice.

1 bunch roughly chopped fresh
flat-leaf or curly parsley

½ cup roughly chopped fresh
mint

1 cup stemmed and chopped
kale

1 mini cucumber, halved
lengthwise, then sliced

½ fennel bulb, core removed,
thinly sliced

1 celery stalk, thinly sliced

1 green onion, thinly sliced

1 can (15 oz) white kidney beans,
drained and rinsed

3 Tbsp extra virgin olive oil

Juice of 1 lemon

1½ tsp sumac

½ tsp sea salt

A few cracks of pepper

⅓ cup chopped toasted or dry-
roasted almonds

⅓ cup pomegranate seeds or
dried cranberries

Breakfast Salad

⊕ ENERGIZE, UPLIFT

PREP TIME: 15 MINUTES **SERVES:** 2–4

Salad may seem like an odd thing to eat for breakfast but, truthfully, many people around the world do eat it for their morning meal. We often think of sweet things when we think of breakfast, but why not get in your rainbow of veggies and fiber early in the day? Plus, salad for breakfast can be refreshing and invigorating. Eating colorful, fresh vegetables, especially in the morning, energizes your brain and body. We have a deep love for Middle Eastern flavors, which is why this salad slightly resembles tabbouleh. The star spice here is sumac, which you can find at most grocery stores—it's a gorgeous reddish purple and tastes lemony. This salad's high fiber content promotes blood sugar balance, which helps keep energy levels and mood stable and steady.

1   Combine the parsley, mint, kale, cucumber, fennel, celery, green onion, and kidney beans in a large bowl.

2   Add the oil, lemon juice, sumac, salt, and pepper, and toss everything together so it's smothered in all the dressing goodness. Top with the almonds and pomegranate seeds.

3   If you would like to reserve some salad for future breakfasts, lunches, or dinners, dress only the portion of the salad you're eating right away. The salad can be kept in the fridge, undressed in an airtight container or bowl, for up to 2 days.

NOTES: 1. *If you want to increase the protein, you can add eggs, tofu, shrimp, chicken, or fish.* **2.** *If you don't have white kidney beans, sub in cannellini or butter beans.*

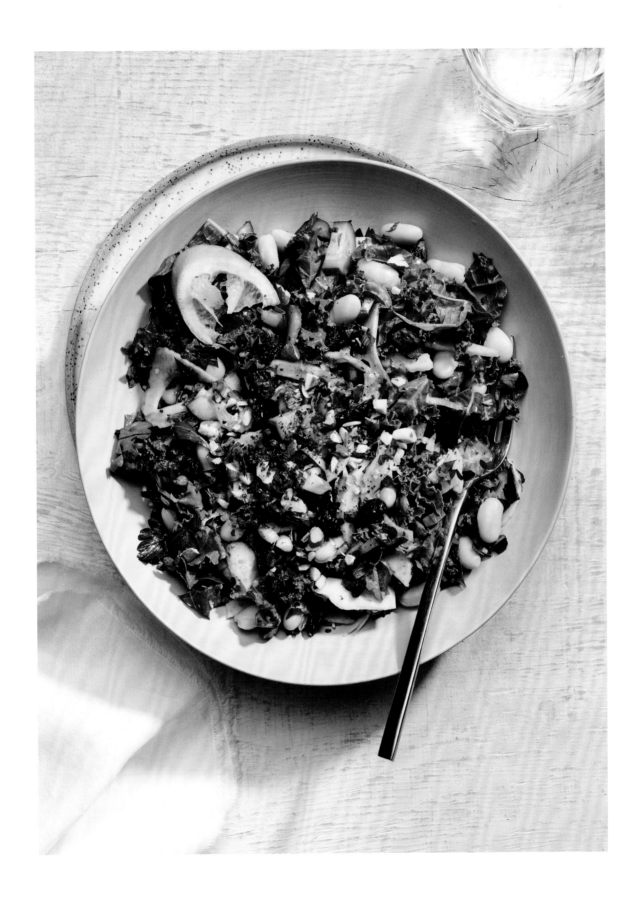

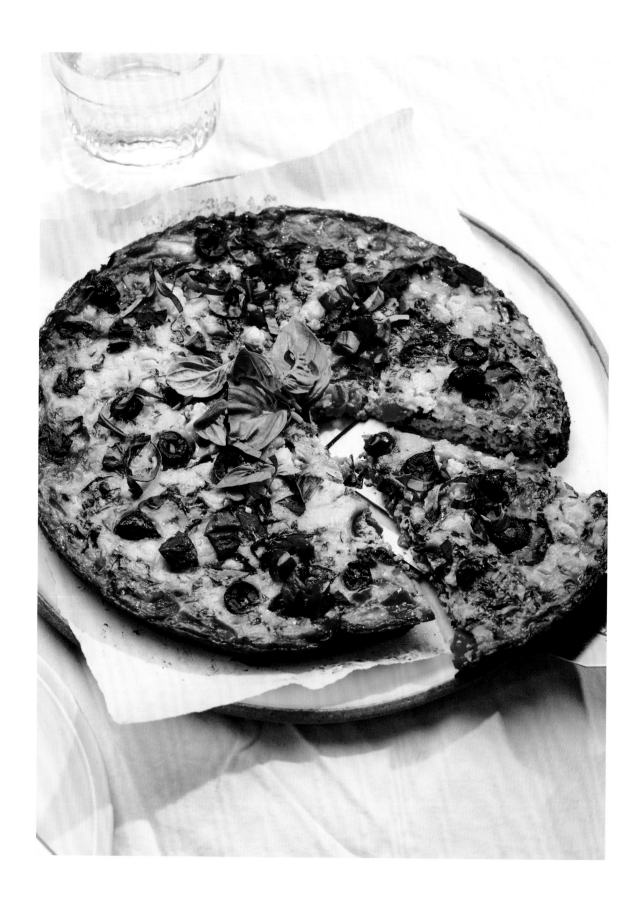

Frittata-za

1 Tbsp extra virgin olive oil

1 cup diced red onion

1 cup diced red bell pepper

6 cherry tomatoes, halved

¼ tsp sea salt, plus a pinch

Pinch of pepper

6 eggs

¼ cup milk of choice

¼ cup roughly chopped kale or spinach leaves

¼ cup crumbled feta

¼ cup fresh basil leaves, roughly torn, plus extra for garnish

6 kalamata olives, pitted and sliced

⊕ **ENERGIZE, FOCUS, UPLIFT**

PREP TIME: 10 MINUTES **COOK TIME:** 20 MINUTES **SERVES:** 2–4

This is our playful and loose take on frittata-meets-pizza. We prepare the veg from scratch here, but if you've got random, leftover cooked veggies sitting in the fridge, you can certainly use those instead. This is a satisfying breakfast filled with protein from the eggs and feta, and fiber from the colorful veggies. Protein helps build feel-good chemicals that keep us happy, alert, and focused.

1 Preheat the oven to 400°F.

2 Place a cast-iron or oven-safe skillet over medium heat, add the oil, and swirl it around to coat the bottom. Toss in the onion, bell pepper, and tomatoes. Season with a pinch each of salt and pepper. Stirring occasionally, cook for 7 minutes or until the veggies are soft and the onion is caramelized.

3 While the veggies are cooking, in a medium bowl, combine the eggs, milk, kale, feta, basil, olives, ¼ tsp salt, and a pinch of pepper.

4 Once the veggies are cooked, pour the egg mixture overtop, help it spread out evenly by shaking the skillet, then leave untouched for about 1 minute.

5 Place in the oven and bake for 10 minutes or until the eggs are cooked through. Sprinkle with basil, if you like.

6 Cut the frittata-za into slices to serve. Store leftovers in an airtight container in the fridge for up to 4 days. Reheat in the oven or toaster oven for a quick breakfast.

1 pint cherry tomatoes

2 tsp extra virgin olive oil

Pinch of sea salt

4 eggs

1 avocado, peeled, pitted, and sliced

1 tsp lemon zest

Squeeze of lemon

½ cup sauerkraut

Pinch of pepper

¼ cup fresh basil leaves, for garnish

Blistered Tomatoes with Jammy Eggs

⊕ ENERGIZE, FOCUS

PREP TIME: 5 MINUTES   **COOK TIME:** 20 MINUTES   **SERVES:** 2

Don't judge us, but . . . we don't love raw tomatoes. Neither of us do. However, when they're roasted, bursting with sweet juice, and blistered—we are here for that. Topped with jammy eggs, avocado, and sauerkraut, this dish checks all the boxes: good protein, healthy fat, colorful fruit (remember, tomatoes are fruit!), and fermented foods. This is the ultimate blood-sugar balancing and gut-nourishing meal to keep energy levels steady for hours and the mind focused.

1   Preheat the oven to 400°F and line a small baking sheet with parchment paper.

2   Spread the tomatoes on the baking sheet, drizzle with the oil, and season with a pinch of salt. Toss to coat.

3   Roast for 15 minutes. You want the tomatoes to be slightly blistered and caramelized at the edges. If they need a little more time, roast for another 3–5 minutes.

4   While the tomatoes are roasting, bring a pot of water to a gentle boil. Using a slotted spoon, carefully lower the eggs into the boiling water. Boil the eggs for 7 minutes. Immediately run the eggs under cold water, peel, and slice the eggs in half.

5   To serve, divide the blistered tomatoes, avocado, and eggs between two plates. Sprinkle with lemon zest, a squeeze of lemon juice, salt, and pepper. Divide the sauerkraut between the plates. Garnish with the basil.

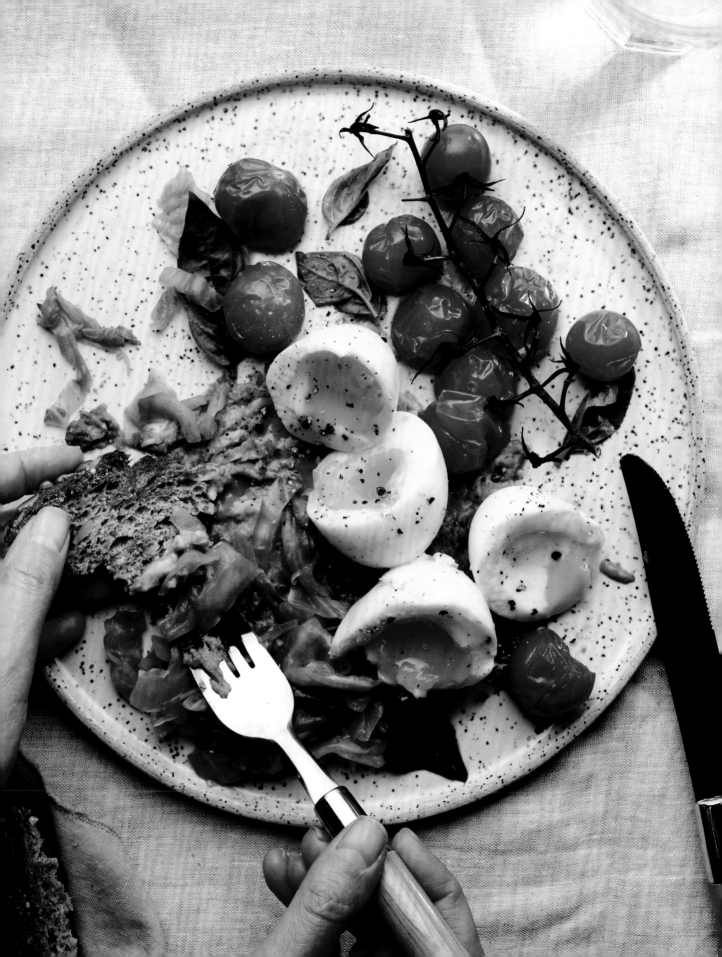

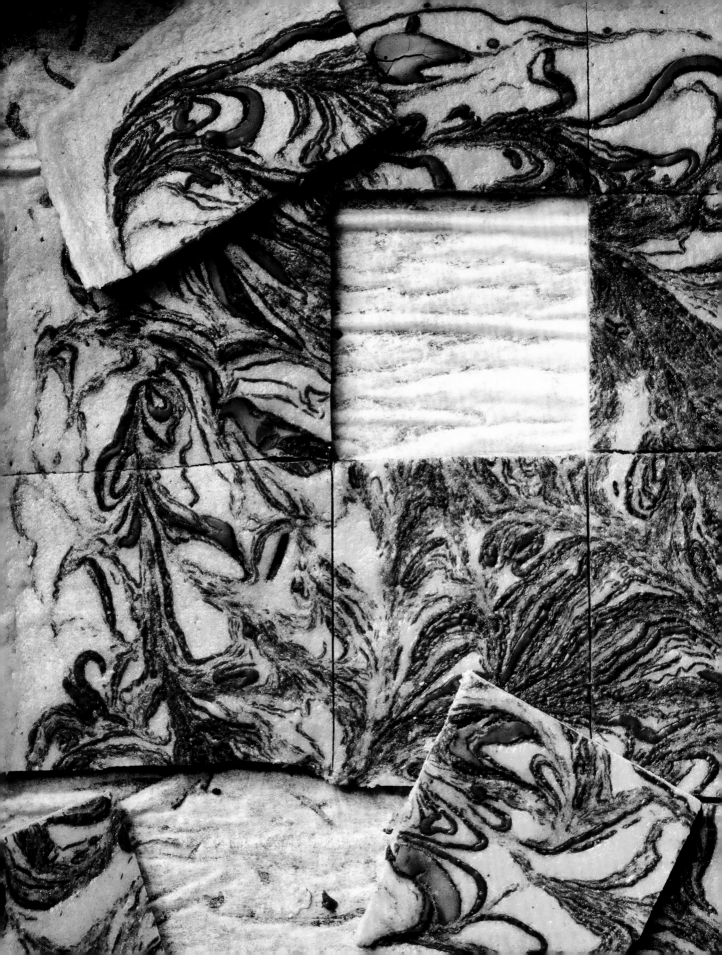

PANCAKES

2 tsp coconut oil or butter

1 cup almond flour

¼ cup arrowroot starch or tapioca starch

½ tsp baking powder

½ tsp baking soda

½ tsp sea salt

3 eggs

2 Tbsp maple syrup

¼ cup milk of choice

CHOCOLATE SWIRL TOPPING OPTION

⅓ cup dark chocolate chips or chopped dark chocolate bar

½ tsp coconut oil

BERRY BURST TOPPING OPTION

½ cup berries of choice (blueberries, blackberries, and/or raspberries)

ADDITIONAL OPTIONAL TOPPINGS

A dollop of yogurt

A drizzle of maple syrup

Sheet-Pan Pancakes

⊕ **ENERGIZE, UPLIFT**

PREP TIME: 15 MINUTES **BAKE TIME:** 20 MINUTES **SERVES:** 4–6

Although we often make classic pancakes at home, we wanted an alternative that would fill up our kids, keep their blood sugar more stable, and deliver fiber to their bodies. These ingredients help the body and mind feel steady, energized, and uplifted, rather than exhausted or foggy. This recipe does all that *and* tastes like a sweet treat, especially with the marbled chocolate swirl on top. You can easily freeze leftovers and toast them up in the morning for quick, yummy breakfasts.

1 Preheat the oven to 350°F. Lightly grease an 11- × 11-inch baking sheet with oil or butter, then place parchment paper on top so it sticks to it.

2 Combine the almond flour, arrowroot starch, baking powder, baking soda, and salt in a medium bowl.

3 Place the eggs, maple syrup, and milk in a separate medium bowl. Mix well.

4 Pour the wet ingredients into the dry and stir until a batter forms. Pour the batter onto the prepared baking sheet and gently shake the baking sheet so that the batter spreads out evenly.

5 **Chocolate Swirl Topping Option:** Melt the chocolate and coconut oil in a double boiler, stirring constantly, until silky. Dollop spoonfuls of the chocolate mixture over the batter, then run a knife or toothpick through it until it looks marbled.

  Berry Burst Topping Option: Scatter the berries over the batter.

6 Bake for 20 minutes or until baked through, firm to the touch, and slightly golden.

7 Slice into squares and enjoy with yogurt, maple syrup, or on their own. Store leftovers in an airtight container in the fridge for up to 5 days. To freeze, put parchment paper between the pancakes, so that you can pull them apart easily once they're frozen. These will keep in the freezer for up to 3 months.

NOTE: *A larger baking sheet will produce thinner pancakes than a smaller one. You may need to bake for less time, so check after 15 minutes.*

High-Fiber Waffles with Berry Syrup

⊕ ENERGIZE, UPLIFT

PREP TIME: 5 MINUTES **COOK TIME:** 20 MINUTES **SERVES:** 2–4

We love a sweet breakfast, but what we love even more is when a sweet breakfast doesn't cause a massive blood sugar spike. We've blended the chia seeds and hemp seeds into the batter, so you won't even know they are there providing you with nourishing fat for brain health and protein for your body to make neurotransmitters—the chemicals that make us feel happy, motivated, focused, and alert.

WAFFLES

½ cup buckwheat flour or spelt flour

½ cup almond flour

⅓ cup hemp seeds

1 Tbsp chia seeds

1 Tbsp coconut sugar

1½ tsp baking powder

¼ tsp sea salt

1 cup milk of choice

1 tsp pure vanilla extract

1 egg or 1 flax egg

3 Tbsp butter or coconut oil, at room temperature, plus more for waffle iron

BERRY SYRUP

1 cup frozen blueberries, raspberries, or strawberries

1 Tbsp maple syrup

ADDITIONAL OPTIONAL TOPPING

Scoop of plain yogurt or dairy-free yogurt

1 Oil and preheat a waffle iron.

2 Put the buckwheat flour, almond flour, hemp seeds, chia seeds, coconut sugar, baking powder, salt, milk of choice, vanilla, egg, and butter in a blender and blend for 20 seconds or until everything is incorporated and smooth.

3 Pour about ½ cup of batter into the waffle iron, depending on its size, close the lid, and let the waffle cook for 2–3 minutes, until golden. Transfer the cooked waffle to a baking sheet or oven-safe dish and place in the oven or toaster oven at 250°F to keep warm until ready to serve. Repeat with the remaining batter.

4 Meanwhile, place the berries and maple syrup in a small pot. Heat on low until the berries are softened. Mash the berries slightly with the back of a spoon, then simmer for 3 minutes. Pour the berry syrup overtop the waffles just before serving. Serve topped with yogurt, if you like.

NOTE: *You can replace the egg with a flax egg. Whisk 1 Tbsp ground flaxseed with 3 Tbsp water, and wait 5–10 minutes until it thickens slightly.*

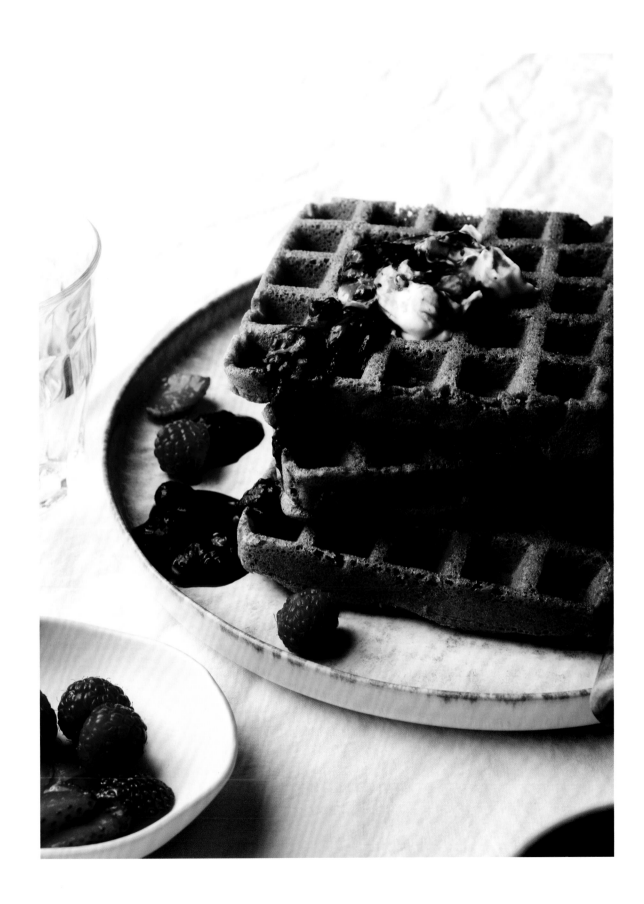

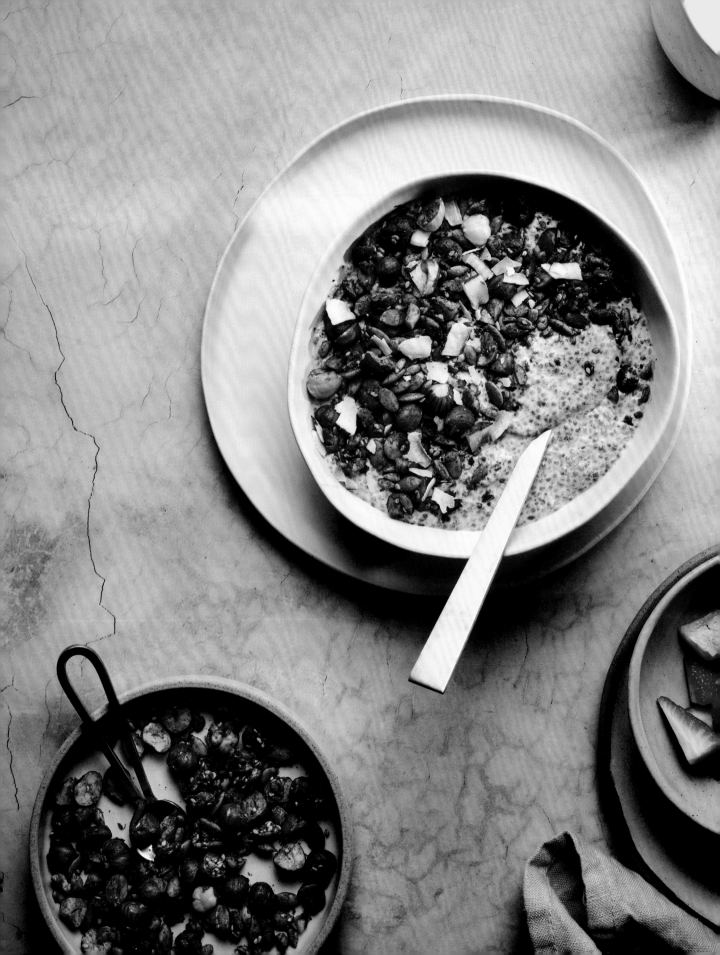

MAPLE BUTTER MOCHA GRANOLA

⅓ cup butter or coconut oil

2 Tbsp maple syrup

2 cups chopped hazelnuts or pecans

½ cup sunflower seeds

½ cup pumpkin seeds

¼ cup sesame seeds

1 Tbsp cacao powder or cocoa powder

1 Tbsp ground decaf coffee

1 Tbsp coconut sugar

Pinch of sea salt

CHIA KEFIR PUDDING

2 cups kefir

⅓ cup chia seeds

1 tsp pure vanilla extract

1 tsp ground cinnamon

Maple syrup to taste

OPTIONAL TOPPINGS

Small handful of fresh berries (blackberries, blueberries, raspberries, or strawberries)

Sliced pear

A few slices of unripe green banana

NOTE: *The chia kefir pudding and granola can be made up to a few days ahead, for easily assembled quick breakfasts.*

Chia Kefir Pudding with Maple Butter Mocha Granola

⊕ **ENERGIZE, FOCUS, UPLIFT**

PREP TIME: 35 MINUTES   **COOK TIME:** 20–25 MINUTES   **SERVES:** 4–6

You may have had chia pudding before, but in this recipe, the addition of kefir lends tanginess, protein, and food for your microbes. The star of the show here is the Maple Butter Mocha Granola (just those words alone make us swoon). Most traditional granolas are filled with sugars, which creates a frenzy for your blood sugar and leaves you feeling unsatisfied a mere hour after eating. We've packed this granola with fatty protein-rich nuts and seeds to keep you feeling full and balanced.

1   Preheat the oven to 350°F and line a baking sheet with parchment paper.

2   In a small pot set over low-medium heat, melt the butter. Pour in the maple syrup and stir until combined, then remove.

3   In a medium bowl, combine the hazelnuts, sunflower seeds, pumpkin seeds, sesame seeds, cacao powder, coffee, coconut sugar, and salt.

4   Pour the maple butter over the dry ingredients and toss to combine. Evenly spread the granola on the prepared baking sheet.

5   Bake for 20–25 minutes—no stirring required. The granola will look brown from the cacao powder and coffee but will not look burned.

6   Remove from the oven and let the granola rest, untouched, for 10 minutes—this will allow it to harden. Set aside or store in an air-tight container at room temperature for up to 1 month (if it lasts uneaten that long!)

7   To make the chia kefir pudding, place the kefir, chia seeds, vanilla, cinnamon, and maple syrup in a medium bowl and mix well. Cover the bowl and place in the fridge for 20 minutes or up to overnight. This will help the pudding thicken.

8   When ready to eat, scoop the pudding into individual bowls, topping each with about ¼ cup of the granola. Top with fresh fruit, if you like. Store any leftover chia pudding in an airtight container in the fridge for up to 5 days.

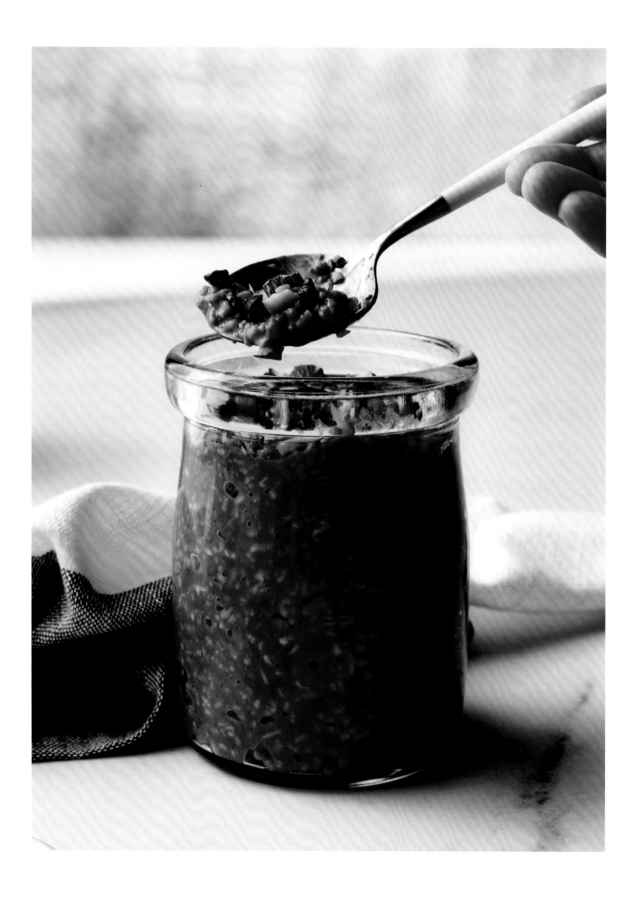

Overnight PB and Chocolate Oatmeal

⊕ **CALM, ENERGIZE, FOCUS**

PREP TIME: 5 MINUTES   **COOK TIME:** OVERNIGHT   **SERVES:** 2

A warming bowl of oatmeal is so nice and calming on a cold morning, when smoothies or eggs just don't cut it. The problem with most people's oatmeal is that they use instant oats, which can cause a major blood sugar spike and crash, prompting a case of brain fog, low energy, and cravings shortly after eating. Here, we use steel-cut oats, which won't spike blood sugar as high and are higher in fiber. We pair them with protein (and chocolate!) for more sustained energy and a balanced mood throughout the day.

½ tsp butter or coconut oil (optional)

½ cup steel-cut oats

½ tsp ground cinnamon

1 heaping tsp cacao powder or cocoa powder

1½ cups water

¼ cup milk of choice (for reheating)

2 Tbsp ground flaxseed

¼ cup hemp seeds or ½–1 scoop protein powder of choice

1 Tbsp peanut butter or almond butter

Maple syrup for drizzling (optional)

¼ cup chopped peanuts, almonds, or pumpkin seeds

1 Tbsp cacao nibs or dark chocolate chips

Small handful of berries of choice

1   Melt the butter in a medium pot set over medium heat. Add the oats and toast them for 1 minute, stirring. Add the cinnamon, cacao powder, and water, bring to a boil, then cover, turn off the heat, allow to cool, and let sit overnight in the fridge.

2   In the morning, transfer about ½ cup of the oatmeal mixture to a clean pot, pour in ¼ cup of milk (or less, if you prefer it thicker), and place over medium heat until warm and gooey. Mix in the ground flaxseed, hemp seeds, peanut butter, and maple syrup, if you like. Top with peanuts, cocoa nibs, and berries.

3   Leftover oatmeal can be stored in an airtight container in the fridge for up to 4 days and reheated in a pot with a little milk for easy, quick breakfasts.

Miso Savory Oats with Soft Boiled Eggs

½ cup steel-cut oats

1½ cups water

Pinch of sea salt

2 eggs

2 tsp white miso paste

1 tsp toasted sesame oil

1 Tbsp toasted sesame seeds

1 Tbsp pumpkin seeds

2 small toasted nori sheets

½ avocado, peeled, pitted, and sliced

Chili oil or hot sauce to taste (optional)

⊕ CALM, ENERGIZE, FOCUS

PREP TIME: 7 MINUTES   **COOK TIME:** 20 MINUTES   **SERVES:** 2

Most people, when they think of oatmeal, think sweet, but a savory oatmeal is just as warming, comforting, hearty, and fiber-rich, leaving you feeling satiated and fueled for hours. Miso adds not only good-for-your-gut ferments, which impacts your every-day brain health and mood, but also that wonderful umami flavor.

1   Place a medium pot over medium heat and add the oats, water, and salt. Cover the pot, bring to a boil, then reduce the heat and simmer for 20 minutes or until the oatmeal is thick-ish.

2   With 10 minutes of cooking time left for the oatmeal, fill a small pot with water, bring to a boil, then gently add the eggs. Cover and reduce the heat to a rapid simmer. Cook for 7 minutes (any longer and the yolks will start to harden). Immediately run the eggs under cold water, peel, and set aside.

3   When the oats are cooked, stir in the miso and sesame oil until well combined.

4   Portion out ¼–½ cup oatmeal into individual bowls, then slice the soft-boiled eggs and place them on top. Sprinkle with sesame seeds, pumpkin seeds, and sliced nori sheets. Arrange the avocado slices overtop, and sprinkle it all with some hot sauce, if you like.

5   If you have leftover oatmeal, store it in an airtight container in the fridge for up to 4 days. Reheat by warming in a pot with a bit of water over low heat.

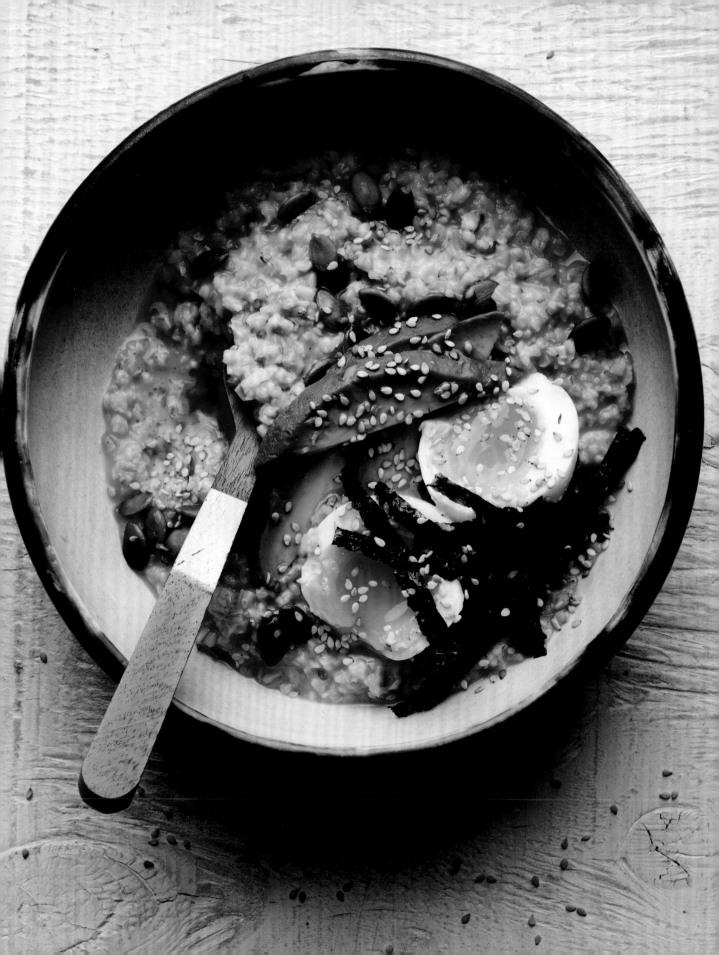

Special Yogurt Bowl

⊕ ENERGIZE, FOCUS, UPLIFT
PREP TIME: 7 MINUTES SERVES: 1

½–¾ cup plain Greek yogurt or dairy-free yogurt (see note)

2 tsp hemp seeds

1 tsp chia seeds or ground flaxseed

1 tsp maple syrup or honey (optional)

½ tsp pure vanilla extract

½ tsp ground cinnamon

2 tsp creamy tahini or nut/seed butter of choice

1 Tbsp sesame seeds or pumpkin seeds

⅓ cup strawberries and blueberries (or any fruit of choice)

1 Tbsp cacao nibs or dark chocolate chips

Tamara: This is "special yogurt" because that is what my youngest, Reese, calls this recipe. He's in love with yogurt, and, funnily enough, my eldest is repulsed by it. I used to make yogurt bowls for myself in the morning, and as soon as I was about to take my first bite, Reese would say, "Can I have that?" and then try to steal my spoon. As someone who was raised as a slight germaphobe, I don't love sharing eating utensils (or bowls, or water bottles, or apple bites . . . ew!). So, I started making him his own yogurt bowl. Every time I made it, he would ask for more and more and more toppings, until it became this Special Yogurt Bowl, the recipe you see before you today. This breakfast will fuel you with protein, probiotic-rich yogurt and polyphenol-rich fruits so you feel energized, balanced, and ready to take on the day.

1 Place the yogurt, hemp seeds, chia seeds, maple syrup, and vanilla in an individual serving bowl and stir well to combine.

2 Sprinkle with cinnamon, drizzle the tahini over, then top with the sesame seeds, berries, and cacao nibs.

NOTE: *We prefer Greek yogurt over other varieties because of the incredible amount of protein it has! And, if you're dairy-free, there are wonderful non-dairy yogurt options for you.*

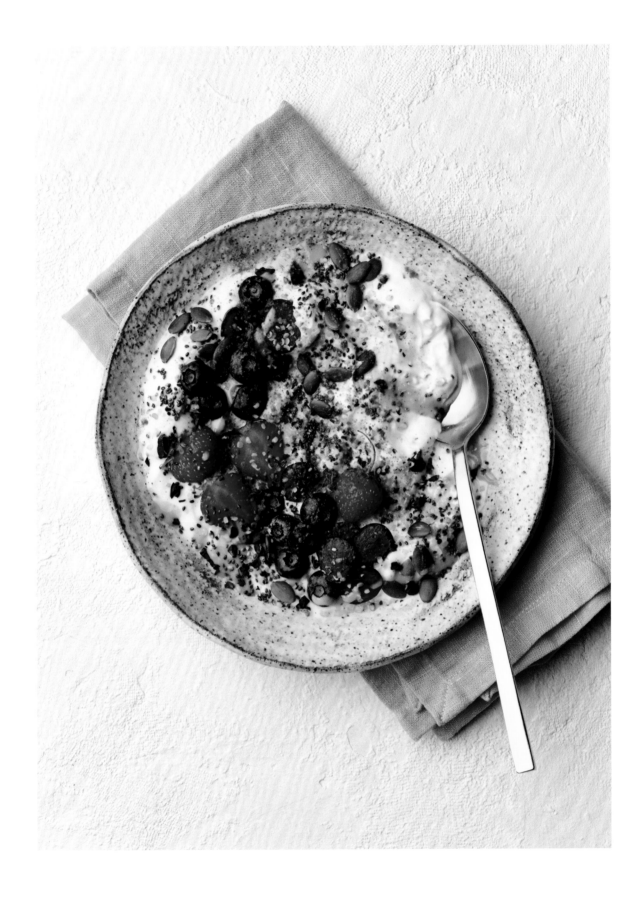

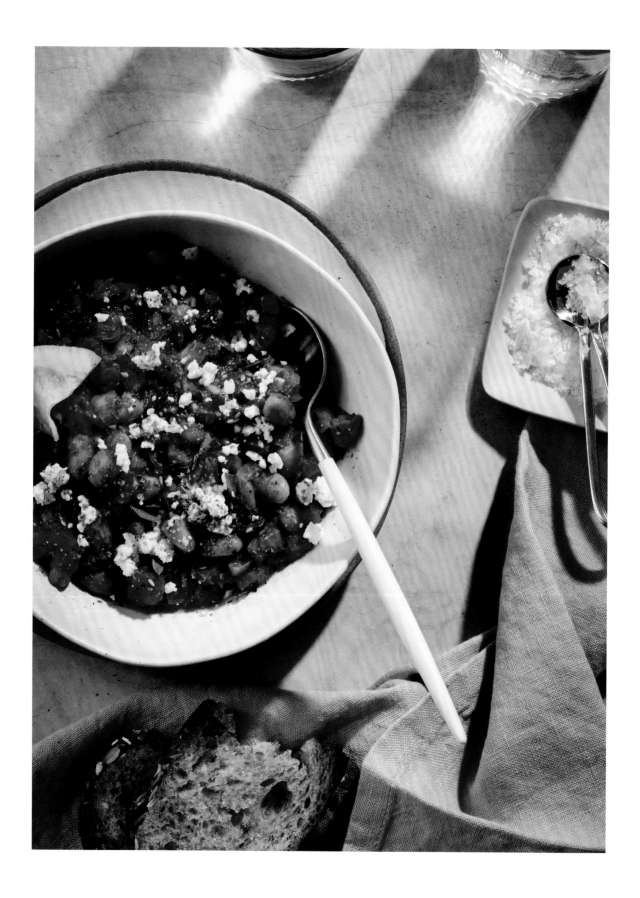

Spiced Tomatoey White Beans

⊕ CALM, ENERGIZE

PREP TIME: 2 MINUTES **COOK TIME:** 20 MINUTES **SERVES:** 2–4

1 Tbsp extra virgin olive oil

1 small red onion, diced

2 garlic cloves, diced

1 tsp sumac

1 tsp paprika

½ tsp ground cumin

½ tsp sea salt

1 can (14 oz) diced tomatoes

1 can (19 oz) cannellini beans
drained and rinsed (see note)

2 cups loosely packed baby
spinach

4 eggs (optional)

Large handful of fresh parsley
or cilantro, roughly chopped

¼ cup slivered or sliced
almonds, toasted

¼ cup crumbled feta (optional)

So many breakfast recipes depend on eggs, especially when you're looking for savory options. But this one provides protein without the eggs, making it a great option whether you're vegan or just can't eat eggs. And, if you love eggs, they're a great addition to this recipe! Inspired by shakshuka, the warm and comforting tomato base infused with sumac, cumin, and paprika is perfect with tender white beans and crunchy almonds, leaving you feeling calm and satiated.

1 Preheat the oven to 375°F.

2 Place a medium oven-safe skillet (we like to use stainless steel or cast-iron) over medium heat, add the oil, and swirl it around to coat the bottom. Once the oil is hot, sauté the onion in it for 3 to 5 minutes, until translucent. Add the garlic, sumac, paprika, cumin, and salt, and sauté for 30 more seconds. Once the spices are fragrant, add the tomatoes, beans, and spinach. Give everything a good stir, then let the mixture simmer for 3 to 4 minutes, until the tomatoes thicken a bit.

3 **If you're not using eggs:** Transfer the skillet to the oven and bake, uncovered, for 10 minutes, or until the liquid is slightly reduced and crusty at the edges.

   If you're using eggs: Use a large spoon to create 4 small wells in the tomato mixture. Crack an egg into each well. Cover the skillet with an oven-safe lid (or use aluminum foil). Bake for 7 minutes or until the egg yolks are cooked to your liking, whether runny or solid.

4 To serve, sprinkle with parsley, almonds, and feta, if you like. Store leftovers in an airtight container in the fridge for up to 4 days.

   NOTE: *If you don't have cannellini, sub navy, white kidney, or great northern beans.*

3 Tbsp extra virgin olive oil,
  divided

1 can (14 oz) pinto beans,
  drained and rinsed

1 tsp chili powder

1 tsp tamari

4 eggs

2 garlic cloves, sliced

1 bunch green kale, stemmed
  and chopped

Sea salt and cracked pepper, to
  taste

OPTIONAL TOPPINGS

Scoop of sauerkraut

Sprouts of choice (sunflower,
  broccoli, alfalfa)

Vermont Mornings Refried Beans

⊕ **ENERGIZE, FOCUS, UPLIFT**

PREP TIME: 5 MINUTES   **COOK TIME:** 15 MINUTES   **SERVES:** 2–4

Sarah: When I was a kid, in the summer we would visit my parents' friends who lived in Vermont. It was still cool in the morning on some of those summer days, and they used to cook this steaming hot breakfast in their cozy kitchen while drinking cups of coffee. It seemed like the perfect slow morning to me. I fell in love with this combo: the runny over-easy eggs, spiced beans, and fresh, bright green kale. With lots of protein and fiber, it'll keep you feeling balanced and focused for hours. Serve with roasted sweet potatoes or toasted sourdough bread for an even more satisfying meal.

1 Place a large skillet over medium heat, add 1 Tbsp of oil, and swirl it around to coat the bottom.

2 Once the oil is hot, add the beans, then stir in the chili powder. Cook for 3 minutes. Add the tamari, stir, and continue to cook for another 2–3 minutes, using the back of a spatula to crush some of the beans.

3 Move the beans to one side of the skillet and add 1 Tbsp of oil. Crack in the eggs. You can cover the skillet with a lid if you like, to help speed up the cooking time. Once the egg whites are solidified and getting crispy at the edges, about 3 minutes, flip the eggs over and cook on the other side for 30 seconds. Portion the hot beans and eggs onto two to four plates, depending on how many people you're serving (feel free to make an extra egg for anyone who wants more).

4 Scrape any extra bits out of the pan, then add the remaining 1 Tbsp oil. Sauté the garlic over medium heat for 30 seconds. Add the kale and cook for 2 minutes or until it's just lightly wilted and bright green. Season with salt and pepper.

5 Serve the hot garlicky kale with the beans and eggs. Top with sauerkraut and sprouts, if you like.

NOTE: *If you don't have pinto beans, you can sub in black beans or a can of refried beans.*

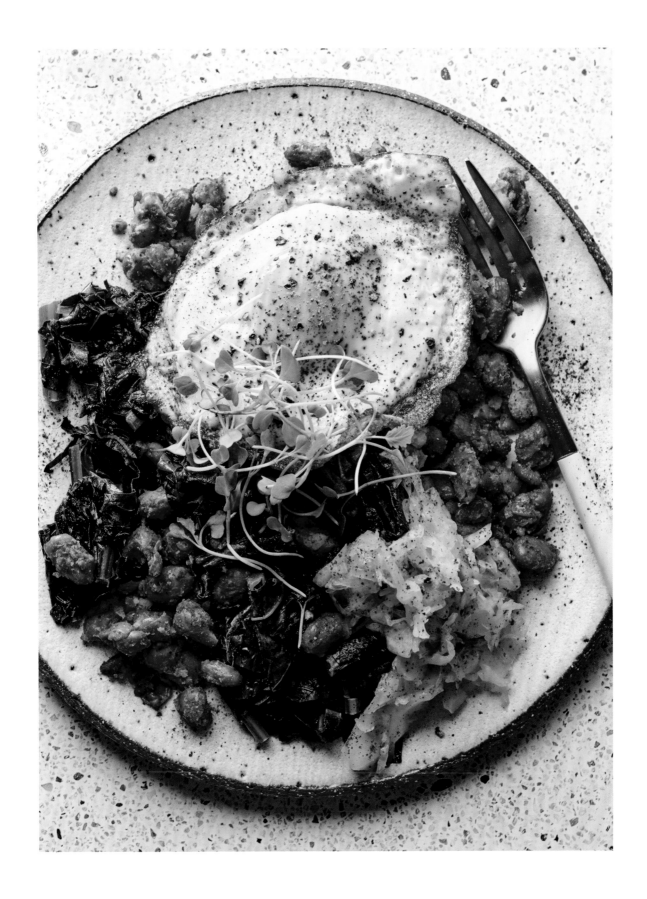

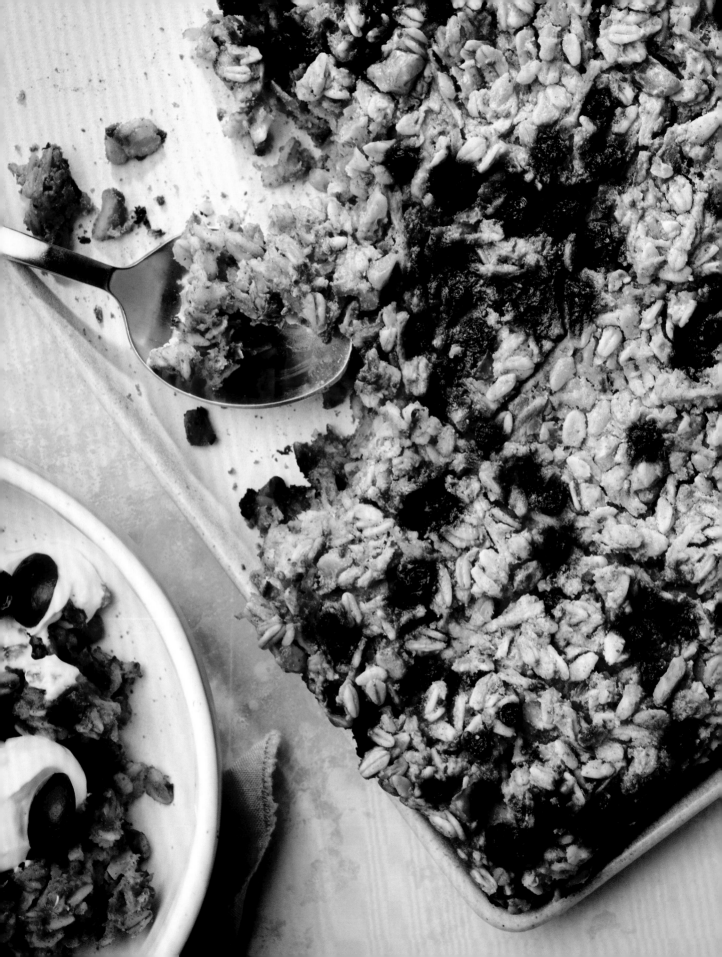

Blueberry Vanilla Yogurt Oatmeal Bake

⊕ CALM, FOCUS, UPLIFT

PREP TIME: 10 MINUTES COOK TIME: 40 MINUTES SERVES: 6

1 Tbsp ground flaxseed

3 Tbsp water

2 cups rolled oats

1 tsp ground cinnamon

½ cup chopped walnuts or pecans

1 Tbsp chia seeds

1 tsp baking powder

¼ tsp sea salt

¼ cup almond butter or nut/ seed butter of choice

1 cup plain Greek yogurt or dairy-free yogurt

1 cup milk of choice

1 tsp pure vanilla extract

2 Tbsp melted coconut oil

1 cup grated apple

½ cup blueberries, fresh or frozen, plus ¼ cup for topping

You can still have your oatmeal and stable blood sugar too (with the addition of protein, fiber, and fat). Yogurt, almond butter, and nuts make a protein-rich breakfast without any eggs required. We love using apple here, for sweetness without added sugars, and chia and flax offer some gentle fiber. You can serve this hot in the winter or chilled in the summer, with a scoop of yogurt for even more probiotics. This breakfast has a nice calming effect on the mind and body and prevents the blood sugar crash, so you can feel clear-headed, full, and stable after you eat it.

1   Preheat the oven to 350°F, and line an 8- × 8-inch baking dish with parchment paper or grease with coconut oil.

2   Stir the ground flaxseed and water together in a small bowl and let sit for 5 minutes while you prepare the other ingredients.

3   In a medium bowl, combine the oats, cinnamon, walnuts, chia seeds, baking powder, and salt.

4   In a large bowl, combine the almond butter, yogurt, milk, vanilla, and melted oil. Add the apple, then whisk in the flaxseed mixture until everything is combined.

5   Fold the dry ingredients into the wet ingredients, along with the blueberries, then give everything a few stirs to combine evenly. Pour into the prepared baking dish, top with additional blueberries, and bake for 40 minutes or until the liquid is absorbed and the mixture is firm to the touch.

6   Scoop out pieces or cut into squares to serve right away. Store leftovers in an airtight container in the fridge for up to 4 days. Reheat in a toaster oven for easy breakfasts.

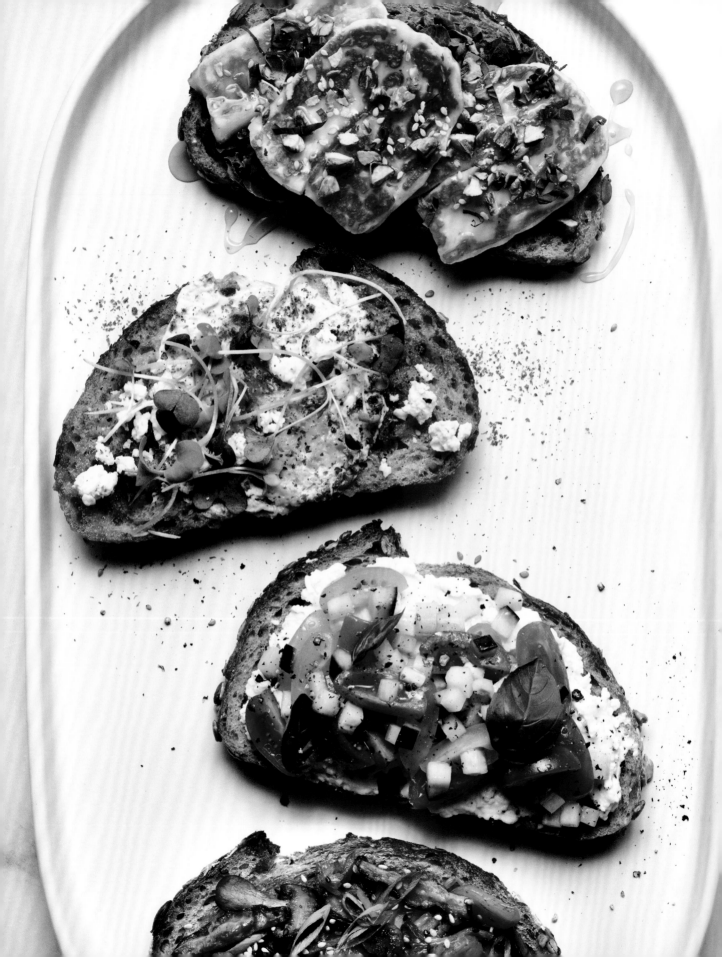

Open Face Sourdough Toasties Four Ways

Sourdough is fermented, which helps the body to digest it; it has fiber, which helps with blood sugar balance; *and* it contains prebiotics, which go on to feed the good bugs in the gut!

+ **Blood Sugar Balancer**
+ **Colorful** + **Fermented**
+ **Fiber-Rich** + **Prebiotic**
+ **Protein-Powered**

4–5 Tbsp cottage cheese

1–2 pieces sourdough bread, toasted

4 cherry tomatoes, halved

3 Tbsp diced cucumber

½ tsp extra virgin olive oil

1 tsp freshly squeezed lemon juice

A few sprigs basil or dill

Sea salt and a few cracks of pepper

Scoop of sauerkraut (optional)

Super Fresh Cottage Cheese Toastie

⊕ **ENERGIZE, UPLIFT**

PREP TIME: 7 MINUTES **SERVES:** 1–2

Cottage cheese has a shocking amount of protein, making it great to eat at any meal but especially the first meal of the day. Protein in the morning helps your brain feel alert and the mind and body feel invigorated. Some cottage cheese has probiotic benefits; try to find a brand that lists live and active cultures on its ingredient list.

1 Spread the cottage cheese on the toasted bread.

2 In a bowl, toss together the tomatoes, cucumber, oil, and lemon juice to mix.

3 Place the vegetable mixture on top of the cottage cheese. Tear fresh herbs and place overtop, then season well with salt and pepper. Enjoy on its own or with a scoop of sauerkraut on the side.

4 If you have leftover vegetable salad, keep it in an airtight container in the fridge for up to 2 days, and eat it as a side or on top of a green salad, cooked grains, or even salmon.

Za'atar Egg-in-a-Hole Toastie

½ tsp butter or extra virgin
    olive oil

1–2 pieces sourdough bread

1–2 eggs

Pinch of sea salt and a few
    cracks of pepper

½ tsp za'atar

1 Tbsp crumbled feta (optional)

4 mint leaves, torn

Broccoli sprouts

Scoop of sauerkraut (optional)

⊕ **FOCUS, UPLIFT**

PREP TIME: 2 MINUTES   **COOK TIME:** 10 MINUTES   **SERVES:** 1–2

Tamara: When I was growing up, egg-in-a-hole was my grandmother's specialty—the runny eggs dripping over the warm, crusty bread was perfection. We're adding a few additional flavors and ingredients, like za'atar, a Middle Eastern spice, that is available at most grocery stores or online. Do not skip this ingredient—it really elevates the toast! It may not always be possible to have fresh broccoli sprouts in the fridge, but if you got 'em, use them here: they are one of the richest sources of the powerful phytonutrient sulforaphane and make a great contribution to this toastie.

1   Heat a small pan over medium heat, add the butter, and swirl it around to coat the bottom.

2   Using a knife, slice a small egg-size circle out of the center of the bread, big and wide enough that an egg can fit in but won't completely fall through.

3   Place the bread in the pan and immediately flip so both sides have a hit of butter on them. Crack the egg into the hole in the bread. Season with salt, pepper, and ½ tsp za'atar.

4   If you like a runnier egg, flip immediately after; if you like a harder yolk wait for a few minutes. Then cook for another 2 minutes on the second side.

5   Take off the heat, transfer the toastie to a plate, and top with feta, mint, and broccoli sprouts. Enjoy on its own or with a scoop of sauerkraut on the side.

Halloumi and Honey Toastie

½ tsp extra virgin olive oil

2–4 thin slices of halloumi cheese

1–2 pieces sourdough bread

Small handful of arugula or baby spinach

Small pinch each of sea salt and pepper

¼ tsp honey

1 Tbsp chopped pistachios

Small sprinkle of toasted sesame seeds

✚ **CALM, UPLIFT**

PREP TIME: 2 MINUTES **COOK TIME:** 8 MINUTES **SERVES:** 1

Is there anything better than the combo of sweet and salty? The saltiness of the halloumi and sweetness of the honey is such a gift to the taste buds. If you don't eat dairy, replacing the halloumi with a dairy-free ricotta, readily found at the grocery store, will be the perfect swap. This is definitely more of an indulgent breakfast that is best to savor on a slow Sunday morning (if you ever have those!), alongside a warm mug of tea or coffee.

1 Place a small pan over medium heat, add the oil, and swirl it around to coat the bottom. Place the halloumi on one side of the pan and the bread on the other side.

2 Flip the bread and halloumi after about 2 minutes. The halloumi should be nicely browned and crisp on the outside, and the bread should be lightly golden and toasted. Fry for another 2 minutes on the other side or until golden and browned, then remove from the heat.

3 To serve, place the bread on a plate, top with arugula, and season with the tiniest pinch each of salt and pepper. Layer on the halloumi, immediately drizzle with honey, and sprinkle with pistachios and sesame seeds.

Kimchi Fried Egg Toastie

⊕ ENERGIZE, UPLIFT

PREP TIME: 2 MINUTES   **COOK TIME:** 12 MINUTES   **SERVES:** 1

2 tsp avocado oil or coconut oil, divided

6 shiitake or cremini mushrooms, sliced

½ tsp tamari

2 Tbsp kimchi

1–2 eggs

1–2 pieces sourdough bread, toasted

1 green onion, sliced (optional)

Pinch of toasted sesame seeds

Kimchi is a traditional Korean dish made of lacto-fermented cabbage and is one the most probiotic-rich fermented foods to eat. These foods assist your gut bugs in making feel-good chemicals like serotonin, which is important for helping you feel stable and optimistic. You can try making it yourself, or, like us, you can buy it in the refrigerated section of your local grocery store. Kimchi can be spicy and sour; it can also have an umami flavor that pairs well with mushrooms and tamari.

1   Place a small pan over medium heat, add 1 tsp of oil, and swirl it around to coat the bottom. Once the oil is hot, add the mushrooms. After a minute, add the tamari, then let the mushrooms cook for 5 minutes, stirring occasionally.

2   Add the kimchi and sauté for only 1–2 minutes to preserve the bacteria cultures. Transfer the mixture to a small plate.

3   Lightly wipe the pan with paper towel, then add the remaining 1 tsp of oil. Once hot, crack the eggs into the pan and cook for 2–3 minutes, then flip.

4   To serve, place the bread on a plate, layer on the kimchi and mushrooms, top with the fried eggs, and sprinkle with green onion and sesame seeds.

Shredded Veggie Fritters with Probiotic Yogurt

⊕ UPLIFT

PREP TIME: 15 MINUTES   COOK TIME: 20 MINUTES
MAKES: ABOUT 11 FRITTERS

4 eggs

1½ cups shredded green cabbage

1 medium carrot, grated

1 cup grated zucchini

1 small yellow onion, grated

½ cup potato starch

1 tsp baking powder

½ tsp sea salt, plus more for serving

Freshly cracked pepper

1 Tbsp extra virgin olive oil or avocado oil

¼ cup plain Greek yogurt or dairy-free yogurt

We are big on eating veggies for breakfast. If you're aiming to eat 30-plus plants a week, sneaking a few veggies into each meal is a great way to reach that goal. Adding more veggies helps populate your gut with good microbes that keep your immune system strong, help with learning, and build your happiness-neurotransmitters. These fritters are wonderfully crisp, with a soft center. Top with yogurt for an extra hit of probiotics. *See photos on pages 80 and 81.*

1   Whisk the eggs in a large bowl.

2   If the cabbage, carrot, zucchini, or onion seem very wet, put them in a sieve or cheesecloth and press out the excess water. Put the veggies, potato starch, baking powder, ½ tsp salt, and pepper in the bowl and stir to combine. You may want to use your hands here to ensure everything is mixed together well.

3   Preheat the oven to 350°F.

4   Place a medium to large cast-iron or nonstick skillet over medium heat, add the oil, and swirl it around to coat the bottom. Once the oil is hot, work in batches (you don't want to overcrowd the pan), scoop in ¼ cup of batter, press down with a spatula to flatten, and cook for about 2–4 minutes per side, until crisp and golden brown. Transfer the cooked fritters to a baking sheet. Repeat with the remaining batter.

5   Bake the fritters for 7–10 minutes until golden.

6   Just before serving, top each fritter with a big dollop of yogurt and sprinkle with a bit of sea salt and pepper. Leftover fritters make great future breakfasts. Keep in an airtight container in the fridge for up to 3 days or freeze in an airtight container for up to 3 months.

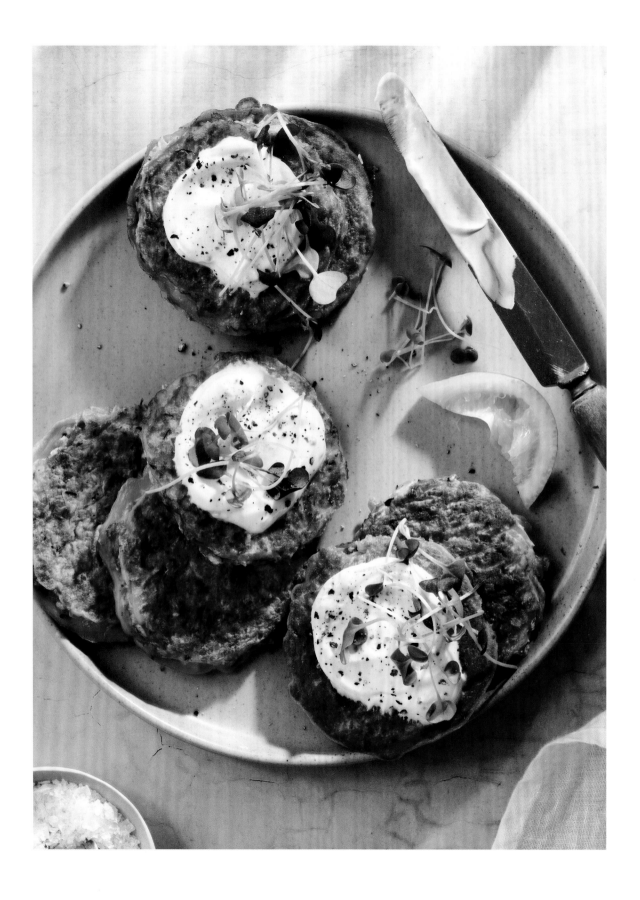

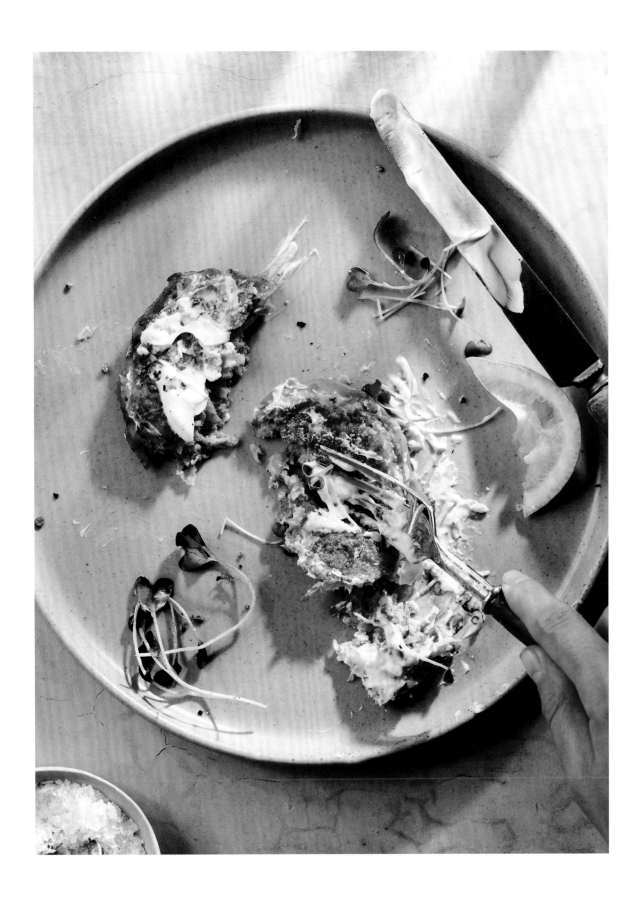

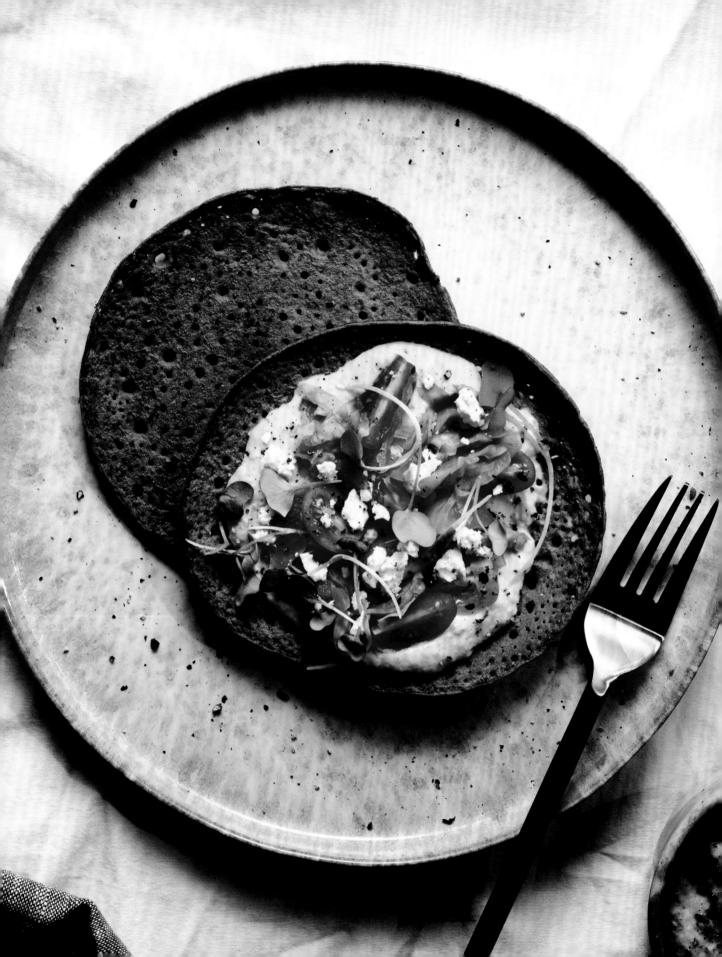

CREPES

1 cup chickpea flour (aka garbanzo flour)

1½ cups water

½ cup loosely packed baby spinach

¼ tsp sea salt

A few cracks of pepper

½ Tbsp extra virgin olive oil, plus more as needed

FILLINGS

A few Tbsp of hummus, pesto, or any spread/dip of choice (see note)

Sliced avocado

Sliced cherry tomatoes

Sauerkraut

Broccoli sprouts

Feta (optional)

Pinch of sea salt and a few cracks of pepper

Chickpea Power Crepes

⊕ CALM, UPLIFT

PREP TIME: 15 MINUTES   **COOK TIME:** 20 MINUTES   **SERVES:** 6

Vibrant green and brimming with fiber from the chickpea flour, these crepes are a wonderful addition to your morning meal. You can get as creative as you like with the fillings, or follow our suggestions below. Freeze any extra crepes for easy breakfasts or use them in place of tortillas or pita bread. Chickpeas are a rich source of B_6 and B_9 (folate), two vitamins needed to improve memory, combat depression, and help build chemicals that make you feel calm, happy, and motivated. Thanks to magnesium-rich spinach, these crepes also help ease stress and overwhelm.

1   Place the chickpea flour, water, spinach, salt, and pepper in a blender or food processor and blend until smooth and bright green. Heat a medium cast-iron or nonstick pan over medium heat. Add ½ Tbsp of oil and swirl it around to coat the bottom.

2   Scoop ¼ cup of chickpea batter into the pan and cook for 1–2 minutes, flipping when little holes start to form in the center. Cook for another 1–2 minutes on the second side. Transfer the cooked crepes to a cooling rack to rest while you make the rest of the crepes. Add more oil to the pan, if needed, to prevent sticking. If the crepes cool down too much, you can pop them in a toaster oven, for a delightfully crisp yet malleable texture.

3   To serve, place a crepe on a plate, spoon hummus or pesto into the center, and spread out evenly. Top with the avocado, tomatoes, sauerkraut, sprouts, feta, salt, and pepper.

4   If you have extra crepes, freeze them in an airtight container or bag, placing parchment paper between each one, for up to 3 months. To reheat, warm in a toaster oven for 1–2 minutes.

NOTE: *You can use our Roasted Root Veggie Hummus on page 90 or Macadamia Parsley Pesto on page 89.*

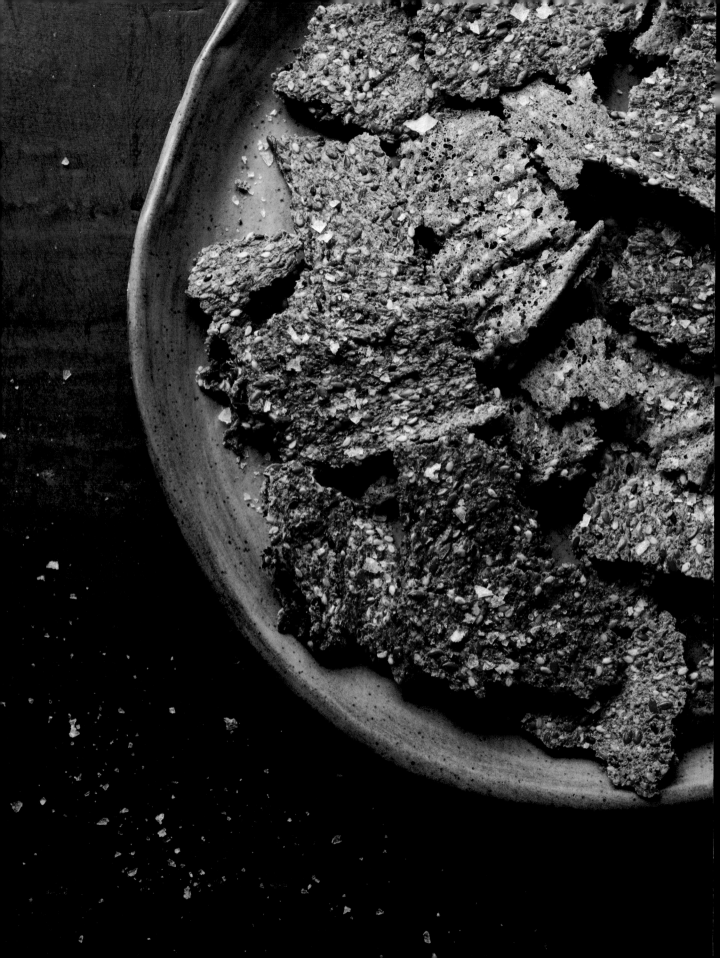

snacks

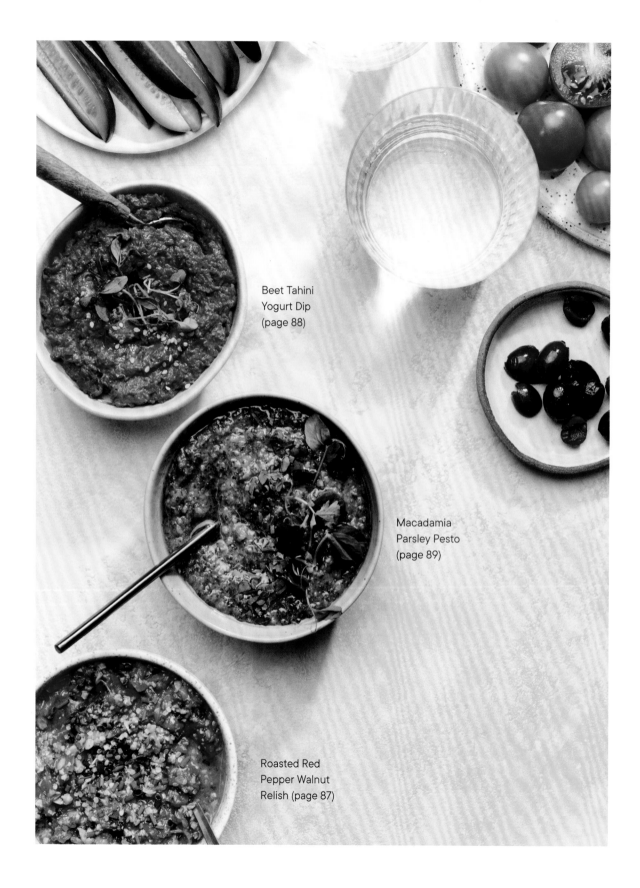

Beet Tahini
Yogurt Dip
(page 88)

Macadamia
Parsley Pesto
(page 89)

Roasted Red
Pepper Walnut
Relish (page 87)

Roasted Red Pepper Walnut Relish

⊕ CALM, UPLIFT

PREP TIME: 10 MINUTES   **COOK TIME:** 5 MINUTES   **SERVES:** 4

½ cup walnuts

2 jarred roasted red bell peppers, roughly chopped

1 small garlic clove, minced

3 Tbsp fresh parsley, chopped

3 Tbsp freshly squeezed lemon juice

1 tsp honey

1 Tbsp extra virgin olive oil

Pinch each of sea salt and pepper

We used to make this recipe for our private cooking clients. That was a decade ago. It's one of those recipes that we forget about, but then every once in a while it resurfaces and we say, "How could we have forgotten about this one?!" So, luckily for you, here it is, forever in this book. You can enjoy it as a dip with crackers or sourdough bread, or even with veggie sticks. Walnuts are the base of the relish—they're a source of omega-3, which is important for overall brain health and especially for alleviating anxiety. Peppers are loaded in B$_6$, helping ease depressive symptoms and create a balanced mood.

1   Preheat the oven to 375°F.

2   Spread the walnuts in a small baking dish and roast for 5 minutes. Check to see that they are lightly browned, and if they aren't toasted yet, give them another minute or two. Once toasted, let the walnuts cool for a few minutes in the dish.

3   Place the roasted red peppers, garlic, parsley, lemon juice, honey, oil, salt, and pepper in a food processor. Add the walnuts and pulse for about 20 to 30 seconds, until everything is roughly chopped. We like to have some chunks of walnuts and roasted red pepper in the mixture, so we don't fully blend it. But, if you prefer a finer chop, you can pulse everything a bit more.

4   Leftovers can be stored in the fridge for up to 2 days. If the mixture separates, give it a good stir before serving.

Beet Tahini Yogurt Dip

⊕ ENERGIZE, FOCUS, UPLIFT

PREP TIME: 7 MINUTES   **COOK TIME:** 25 MINUTES   **SERVES:** 4

1⅓ cups cubed peeled red beets (about 2 medium)

2 tsp extra virgin olive oil

Sea salt, to taste

Pinch of pepper

¼ cup tahini

½ cup plain Greek yogurt or dairy-free yogurt

2 Tbsp freshly squeezed lemon juice, plus more to taste

1 small garlic clove, minced

1–3 Tbsp water

Sprinkle of sumac, for garnish (optional)

Sprinkle of sesame seeds, for garnish (optional)

Drizzle of extra virgin olive oil, for garnish (optional)

This dip has just about everything: probiotics from yogurt and fiber from beets to support your microbiome. Tahini provides healthy fat and additional protein, and we love how it tastes when paired with tangy yogurt and zesty lemon—it's a rich, creamy dip with the perfect amount of tartness and bite. Fat, fiber, and protein all support blood sugar balance, making this a filling and energizing snack to eat, especially during that 3 p.m. crash.

1   Preheat the oven to 375°F.

2   Spread the beets in a baking dish and rub with the oil, salt, and pepper. Roast for about 25 minutes, until the beets are tender.

3   Place the roasted beets, tahini, yogurt, lemon juice, and garlic in a food processor. Pulse a few times to combine. If the mixture seems too thick, gradually add the water, 1 Tbsp at a time, blending between additions. You're looking for a smooth and creamy consistency. Taste and add more lemon or sea salt, if you like.

4   Garnish with the sumac and sesame seeds, if you like, and a small drizzle of extra virgin olive oil.

NOTE: *For a quicker version of this recipe, buy cooked beets or steam the beets instead of roasting them.*

¾ cup macadamia nuts (see note)

1½ cups roughly chopped fresh parsley

½ cup extra virgin olive oil

3 tsp freshly squeezed lemon juice, plus more to taste

1 small garlic clove, minced

¼ tsp sea salt, plus more to taste

Pinch of pepper, plus more to taste

Macadamia Parsley Pesto

✚ **ENERGIZE, FOCUS**

PREP TIME: 10 MINUTES   **COOK TIME:** 3–5 MINUTES   **SERVES:** 4

We love making variations on classic basil pesto, because really there is a whole world of other herbs that are just as delicious as basil. Parsley tastes uplifting and fresh in this pesto and pairs well with the subtle sweetness of toasted nuts. We recommend using macadamia nuts because they are so creamy and reminiscent of parmesan, there's no need to add any cheese to this recipe. The combination of fresh parsley and macadamia nuts supports blood sugar balance and stable energy, helping you feel full for hours after eating. Serve this as a dip with veggie sticks, crackers, or sourdough bread, or even toss with noodles of your choice.

1 Preheat the oven to 375°F.

2 Spread the macadamia nuts in a small baking dish and roast for 3–5 minutes, until lightly toasted.

3 Transfer the toasted macadamia nuts, along with the parsley, oil, lemon juice, garlic, salt, and pepper, to a food processor and pulse several times, until the mixture is chunky. Blend for longer if you prefer a smoother texture for your pesto. Taste and season with salt, pepper, or more lemon juice, if needed.

4 Store in an airtight container in the fridge for up to 5 days or in the freezer for up to 2 months.

NOTE: *If you don't have macadamia nuts, you can sub in almonds or walnuts.*

2 carrots, peeled and cut
in ½-inch pieces (heaping
½ cup)

1 parsnip, peeled and cut
in ½-inch pieces (heaping
½ cup)

2 tsp extra virgin olive oil,
plus more as needed and
for drizzling

4 large garlic cloves

1½ cups cooked chickpeas or
1 can (14 oz) chickpeas,
drained and rinsed

2 Tbsp tahini

1 Tbsp freshly squeezed lemon
juice

½ tsp sea salt

6–8 Tbsp water

Sprinkle of paprika, for garnish
(optional)

Handful of fresh parsley,
chopped, or sprouts for
garnish (optional)

Roasted Root Veggie Hummus

⊕ ENERGIZE, FOCUS, UPLIFT

PREP TIME: 10 MINUTES **COOK TIME:** 35 MINUTES **SERVES:** 6

Sarah: We always have hummus in my house—it really is my go-to snack. I got really tired of store-bought hummus, so I now whip up a batch of hummus every week (of course, in a time crunch, I'll grab it from the store). It's so much more flavorful and nutritious when you make it yourself. With this version of hummus, you'll get a punch of fiber from the carrots, parsnips, tahini, and creamy roasted garlic. It's a super easy way to add more colors and plants into your diet, helping to immediately invigorate the body and mind.

1 Preheat the oven to 375°F and line a baking sheet with parchment paper.

2 Toss the carrots and parsnips with 2 tsp of oil and spread on the prepared baking sheet. Rub the garlic cloves with oil and place in a corner of the baking sheet.

3 Roast for 20 minutes, then give the carrots and parsnips a stir. Remove the garlic cloves from the oven at the 20-minute mark; they'll be nice and soft. Roast the carrots and parsnips for another 10 minutes or until they are starting to caramelize at the edges.

4 Transfer the roasted vegetables and garlic to a food processor along with the chickpeas, tahini, lemon juice, salt, and a few Tbsp of water and blend for about 1 minute, until the mixture is smooth and creamy. Scrape down the sides of the food processor with a spoon or spatula to make sure everything is blended nicely. If the mixture is too thick, you can gradually add more water, 1 Tbsp at a time, and blend again.

5 To serve, place the hummus in a bowl and drizzle oil overtop. Sprinkle with paprika and parsley, if you like. Store any leftovers in an airtight container in the fridge for up to 5 days.

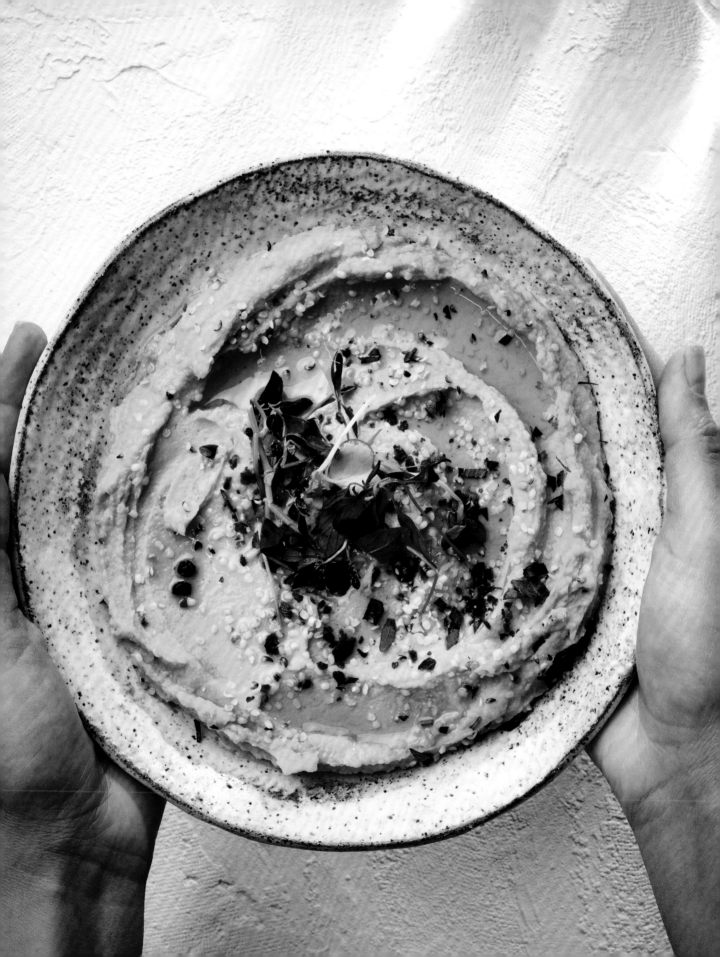

2 apples of choice, cored,
    and cut in thin wedges

2 Tbsp creamy tahini

¼ tsp ground cinnamon

½ tsp cacao powder

1 Tbsp hemp seeds

1 Tbsp sesame seeds

Small handful of walnuts,
    roughly chopped

Apple Slices with "The Works"

⊕ **ENERGIZE**

PREP TIME: 10 MINUTES **SERVES:** 2–4

Tamara: This is one of my favorite 3 p.m. snacks, and it's especially wonderful if you have children who seem to have stomachs that are bottomless pits. Simply lay sliced apples out on a serving platter and be as creative as you like sprinkling your choice of toppings over. The toppings in the recipe happen to be those we personally enjoy the most, but this recipe can be easily adapted to what you have on hand in your kitchen. Pairing fruit with tahini, hemp seeds, sesame seeds, and walnuts creates a stabilizing effect on your energy levels, so you feel satiated after eating and for hours to come.

1 Arrange the apple slices on a plate.

2 Drizzle tahini on top, then sprinkle with cinnamon and cacao powder, followed by the hemp seeds, sesame seeds, and walnuts. Or get creative using toppings of your choice. Enjoy immediately.

1 head garlic

2 Tbsp extra virgin olive oil, plus more for drizzling

20 kalamata olives, pitted and roughly chopped

5 sun-dried tomatoes, roughly chopped

½ tsp Dijon mustard

FOR SERVING (OPTIONAL)

Crackers

Sourdough bread

Veggie sticks

Olive Tapenade

⊕ ENERGIZE, FOCUS

PREP TIME: 5 MINUTES **COOK TIME:** 30 MINUTES **SERVES:** 4

Olives and roasted garlic make the perfect pair: slightly sweet and salty. This tapenade is delicious served with crackers or crusty bread, and you'll get lots of prebiotic fuel from the garlic and nourishing monounsaturated fat from the olives, creating stable energy immediately after eating. We love to spread this tapenade on our Chickpea Flour Crackers (page 106).

1 Preheat the oven to 400°F and line a small baking sheet with parchment paper.

2 Cut about ¼-inch off the top of the head of garlic—this will make it a lot easier to squeeze out the garlic cloves once it's roasted. Place the head of garlic on the prepared baking sheet, drizzle with olive oil, and roast for 30 minutes or until soft.

3 Place 2 Tbsp oil, olives, sun-dried tomatoes, and Dijon mustard in a food processor. Squeeze the soft roasted garlic into the food processor. Pulse everything together a few times, until you have a nice, chunky texture. If you prefer a smoother texture, you can blend it for longer.

4 Serve with crackers, sourdough bread, and/or veggie sticks. Store leftovers in an airtight container in the fridge for 1 week or in the freezer for up to 3 months.

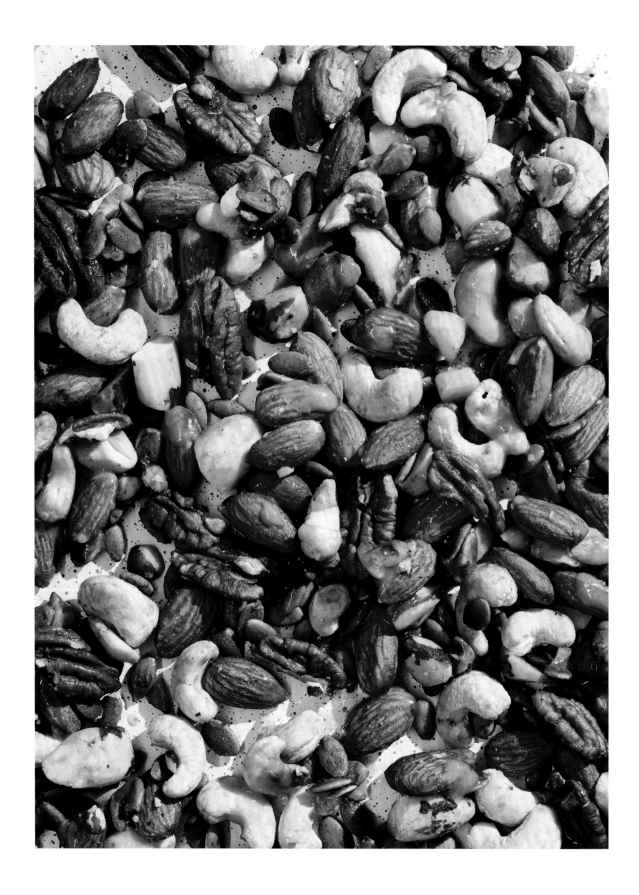

Miso Maple Sticky Nuts

+ Blood Sugar Balancer
+ Fermented + Fiber-Rich
+ Healthy Fats + Prebiotic

⊕ ENERGIZE, UPLIFT

PREP TIME: 10 MINUTES **COOK TIME:** 15–20 MINUTES

MAKES: ABOUT 4½ CUPS

Nut clusters are a great snack midday when you're feeling a blood sugar low, but they're also wonderful toppers on salads or any dish that needs a little bit of oomph. Roasted nuts are already naturally sweet and earthy, but glazing them with miso and maple takes these from good to amazing.

1 cup almonds

1 cup cashews

1 cup pecans

1 cup pumpkin seeds

½ cup chopped Brazil nuts

3 Tbsp maple syrup

3 Tbsp water

2 Tbsp white miso paste

1 tsp butter or coconut oil

⅛ tsp sea salt, plus more to taste

Pinch of cayenne (optional)

1 Preheat the oven to 350°F and line a baking sheet with parchment paper.

2 Place the almonds, cashews, pecans, pumpkin seeds, and Brazil nuts on the prepared baking sheet and roast for 10–15 minutes, until they are lightly golden brown. Keep an eye on them so they don't burn.

3 As the nuts are roasting, heat the maple syrup and water in a small pot set over medium heat until bubbling. Let the mixture bubble until it slightly thickens and stir occasionally; this takes about 6–8 minutes. Turn off the heat and whisk in the miso, butter, salt, and cayenne.

4 Remove the nuts from the oven and pour the maple mixture overtop the nuts on the baking sheet. Stir well to coat all the nuts. Return the nuts to the oven for 3–5 minutes. Remove from the oven and sprinkle a bit more sea salt overtop. Allow the nuts to cool for 10 minutes, then enjoy.

5 Store in an airtight container at room temperature for up to 2 days or in the fridge for up to 1 week.

½ cup ground flaxseed

3 Tbsp flaxseeds

3 Tbsp sesame seeds

1 Tbsp poppy seeds

½ tsp sea salt

¾ cup boiling water

Sprinkle of flakey sea salt

Easy Seedy Flax Crackers

⊕ ENERGIZE, FOCUS

PREP TIME: 25 MINUTES **COOK TIME:** 30 MINUTES **SERVES:** 4

Homemade seed crackers have become an incredibly popular recipe on the internet. This is our take on them. The flax and water act like a natural binder to help keep these crackers structurally sound. They're packed with fiber and healthy fats, making them a good snacking cracker that won't mess with your blood sugar and will keep you feeling steady and balanced.

1 Combine the ground flaxseed, flaxseeds, sesame seeds, poppy seeds, and salt in a bowl. Pour the boiling water over the mixture, mix well, and let sit for 20 minutes.

2 Preheat the oven to 350°F and line a baking sheet with parchment paper.

3 Spread the seed mixture on the prepared baking sheet. Use the back of a spoon or a spatula to smooth it out as evenly as possible, about ⅛-inch thick.

4 Bake for 30 minutes, until golden brown and crisp but not burned-looking. Sprinkle with a pinch of flakey sea salt.

5 Allow to cool fully, then break up the slab into your desired shapes and sizes. Store in an airtight container at room temperature for up to 2 weeks.

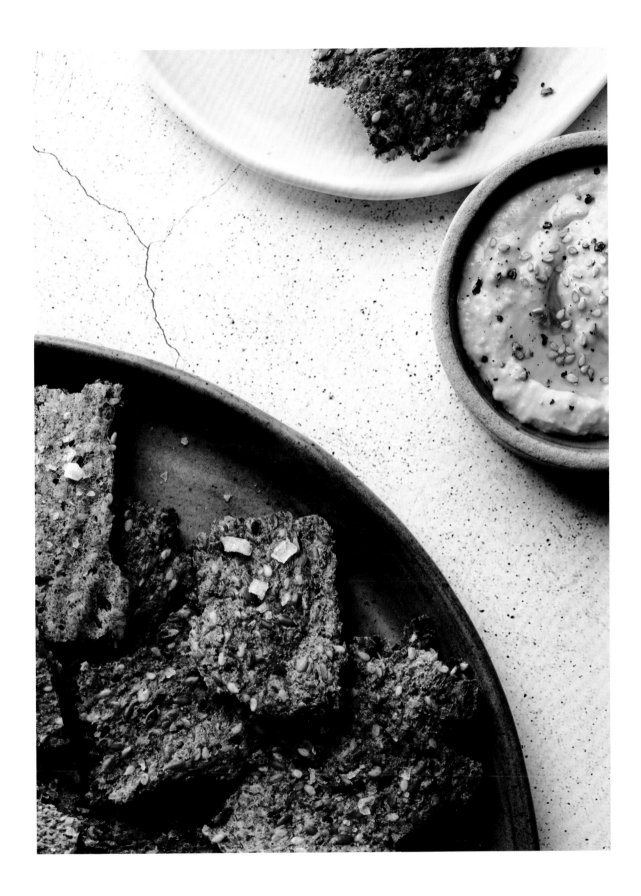

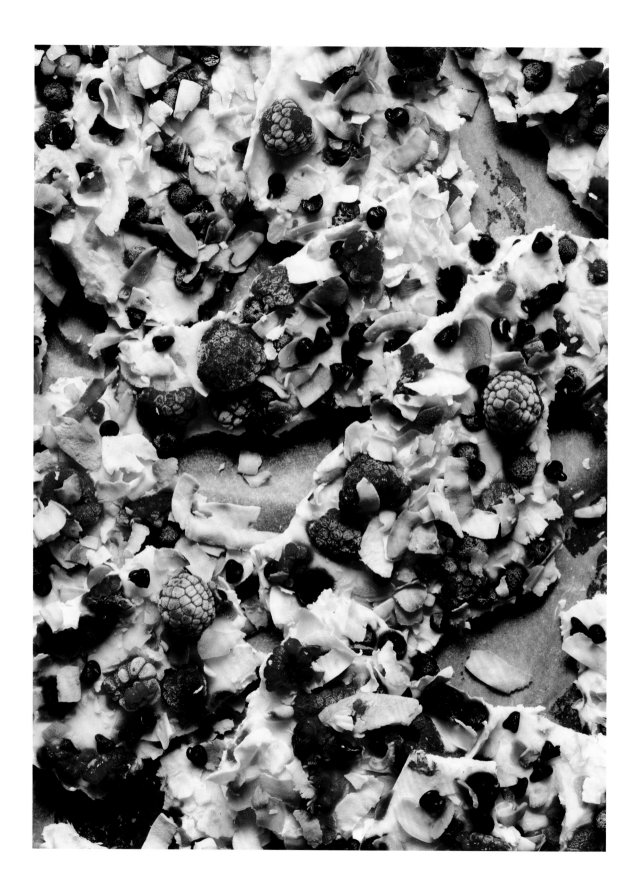

Frozen Yogurt Berry Bark

2 cups plain Greek yogurt or dairy-free yogurt

1 tsp pure vanilla extract

3 Tbsp maple syrup or honey

½ cup toasted almonds, roughly chopped

1½ cups mixed berries (blueberries, raspberries, blackberries), fresh or frozen

½ cup roughly chopped dark chocolate or dark chocolate chips

¼ cup thick coconut chips

Drizzle of honey (optional)

⊕ **ENERGIZE, UPLIFT**

PREP TIME: 10 MINUTES **FREEZER TIME:** 3–4 HOURS **SERVES:** 6–8

This is a great pick-me-up recipe, whether it's enjoyed as a snack or a dessert. The protein-rich yogurt and polyphenol-rich fruits help your body make feel-good neurotransmitters to uplift you, and the magnesium-rich chocolate helps you feel calm. Simply spread yogurt out on a baking sheet and go nuts with the toppings you love.

1 In a medium bowl, combine the yogurt, vanilla, and maple syrup, mixing well.

2 Line a large baking sheet with parchment paper and evenly spread the yogurt mixture on it, making it as thin as you can. Cascade the almonds, berries, chocolate, and coconut chips overtop, then gently press them in to ensure they stick. Drizzle honey overtop if you'd like to add extra sweetness.

3 Place in the freezer for 3–4 hours. Once completely frozen, break into jagged pieces. Store in an airtight container in the freezer for up to 1 month.

Nori Snack Rolls with Avocado and Kimchi

⊕ ENERGIZE, FOCUS, UPLIFT
PREP TIME: 5 MINUTES **SERVES:** 2

2 large nori sheets, ideally
   roasted

1 cup cooked brown rice

1 small avocado, peeled, pitted,
   and thinly sliced

1 small carrot, cut into thin
   matchsticks

1/4 cucumber, cut into thin
   matchsticks

2 Tbsp kimchi

1 Tbsp sesame seeds

1 Tbsp coconut aminos or
   tamari (optional)

This recipe is inspired by Japanese nori rolls. Nori is probably the easiest seaweed to integrate into your diet—you can find it in most grocery stores, and you don't have to do anything to prepare it. Seaweed is an incredible source of minerals, and paired here with avocado means you'll also get lots of nourishing fat to support your hormones and neurotransmitters (feel-good chemicals). For this recipe, we recommend using nori that's been roasted, as it really elevates the flavor. If you don't like spicy kimchi, look for a mild version.

1   Place the nori sheets on a flat clean surface, such as a large cutting board. Carefully spread ½ cup of brown rice on each sheet.

2   Place slices of avocado, carrot and cucumber in a row down the center of each piece of nori, dividing it evenly between the two sheets. Top each row of avocado with 1 Tbsp of kimchi, spreading it out so it lies flat. Sprinkle the sesame seeds overtop.

3   Starting at one edge, roll up the filled nori sheet until you have a neat log. Repeat with the second nori sheet. Eat the roll like a handroll, or slice it into smaller pieces with a serrated knife. If you like, serve with coconut aminos or tamari for dipping.

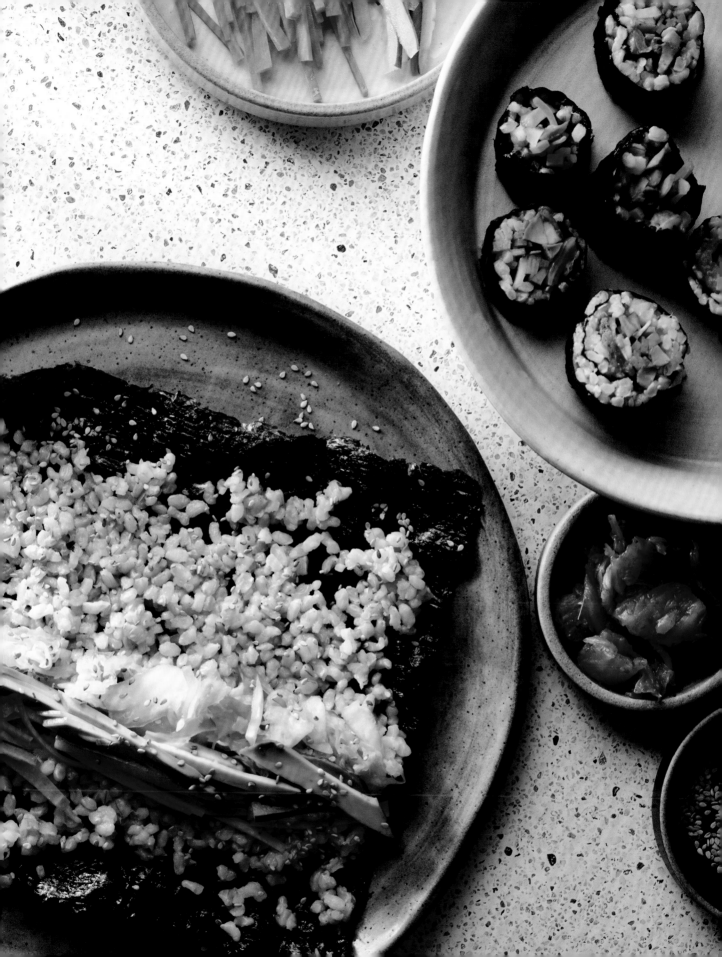

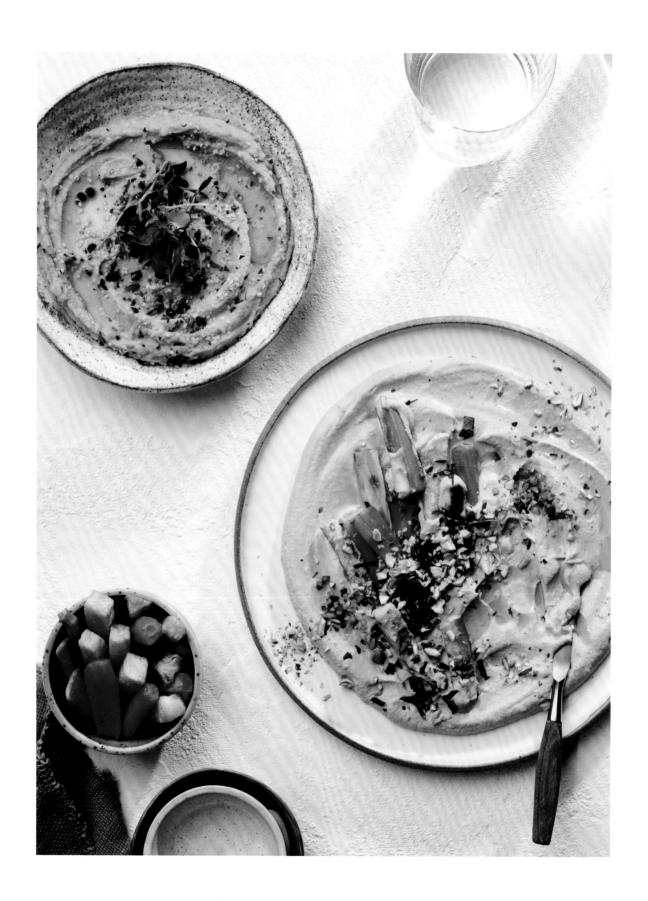

HERBY CASHEW DIP

1½ cups raw cashews

1 head garlic

1 tsp extra virgin olive oil

1¼ cups roughly chopped fresh
parsley and/or basil

¾ tsp sea salt

4 Tbsp freshly squeezed lemon
juice

1 cup water

ROASTED VEGGIE STICKS

2 carrots, peeled and cut in
2-inch-long spears

2 yellow or red beets, peeled
and cut in 2-inch-long spears

1 small jicama or turnip, peeled
and cut in 2-inch-long spears

2 broccoli stalks, peeled and cut
in 2-inch-long spears

3 tsp extra virgin olive oil

¼ tsp sea salt

Pinch of pepper

Herby Cashew Dip with Roasted Veggie Sticks

⊕ ENERGIZE, FOCUS

PREP TIME: 45 MINUTES **COOK TIME:** 40 MINUTES **SERVES:** 4-6

Combining cashews and fresh herbs makes a wonderfully creamy dip that offers healthy, anti-inflammatory monounsaturated fat and protein—the key nutrients to support your energy and mood.

1 To make the herby cashew dip, place the cashews in a large heat-safe bowl and pour boiling water overtop to completely submerge them. Soak for 30 minutes.

2 Preheat the oven to 400°F and line a baking sheet with parchment paper.

3 Slice about ¼-inch off the top of the head of garlic, so it will be easy to squeeze out the garlic once it's roasted. Place in a small baking dish, drizzle with a little oil, and roast for 25–30 minutes, until softened.

4 Spread the sliced carrots, beets, jicama, and broccoli stalks on the prepared baking sheet and use your hands to rub with the oil, salt, and pepper. Make sure the vegetables aren't overcrowding the sheet—this will help them crisp at the edges (you can use two baking sheets if you need more space). Roast for about 20 minutes, then give everything a stir. Roast for another 5–10 minutes, until the vegetables are starting to crisp at the edges.

5 While the vegetables are roasting, drain the cashews in a colander and rinse them. Transfer the soaked cashews to a food processor. Squeeze the soft roasted garlic into the food processor. Add the parsley, basil, salt, lemon juice, and water. Blend until you have a smooth and creamy mixture. Scrape the mixture from the sides of the food processor a few times and continue to blend until the mixture is well combined.

6 Pour the cashew dip into a bowl and serve with the roasted veggie sticks. Store leftovers in an airtight container in the fridge for up to 4 days.

GORP Cookies

⊕ ENERGIZE, UPLIFT

PREP TIME: 5 MINUTES **COOK TIME:** 15 MINUTES **MAKES:** 14 COOKIES

1 egg

1 cup tahini or nut/seed butter of choice (see note)

¼ cup maple syrup

1 cup unsweetened shredded coconut

½ cup dried cranberries (see note)

¼ cup raisins

½ cup cacao nibs or dark chocolate chips

¼ cup raw pumpkin seeds

¼ cup raw sunflower seeds

½ tsp baking soda

Pinch of sea salt

This is an awesome trail mix cookie that's a million times better than good old raisins and peanuts (GORP). Well loved by our private chef clients, it's based on a recipe that a fellow holistic nutritionist, Alexis Nilsen, originally developed. We've created many variations of these cookies over the years, because it's easy to swap ingredients based on what you have on hand or what you like. Thanks to the tahini (or nut butter) and the many seeds, these cookies are the perfect snack with protein and fat to keep you full for longer and energized whether you're taking them on a hike or just need a snack at home.

1   Preheat the oven to 350°F and line a baking sheet with parchment paper.

2   Whisk the egg in a bowl, then stir in the tahini and maple syrup. Add the coconut, cranberries, raisins, cacao nibs, pumpkin seeds, sunflower seeds, baking soda, and salt and stir to combine (it will be a very sticky dough).

3   Using your hands, form the dough into balls a bit larger than a golf ball, and gently flatten. Place them on the baking sheet, about 1-inch apart. Bake for 15 minutes, or until slightly golden on top.

4   Remove from the oven and let cool for 10–15 minutes before removing from the baking sheet. Allow them to cool completely before packing into a storage container. You can store at room temperature for up to 2 days and then in the fridge for up to 1 week.

NOTES: 1. *For the best texture, we recommend using a tahini or nut butter that leans on the liquidy side, so don't use bottom-of-the-jar nut butter that's hardened up.* **2.** *Feel free to use different dried fruit, such as goji berries or dried cherries.*

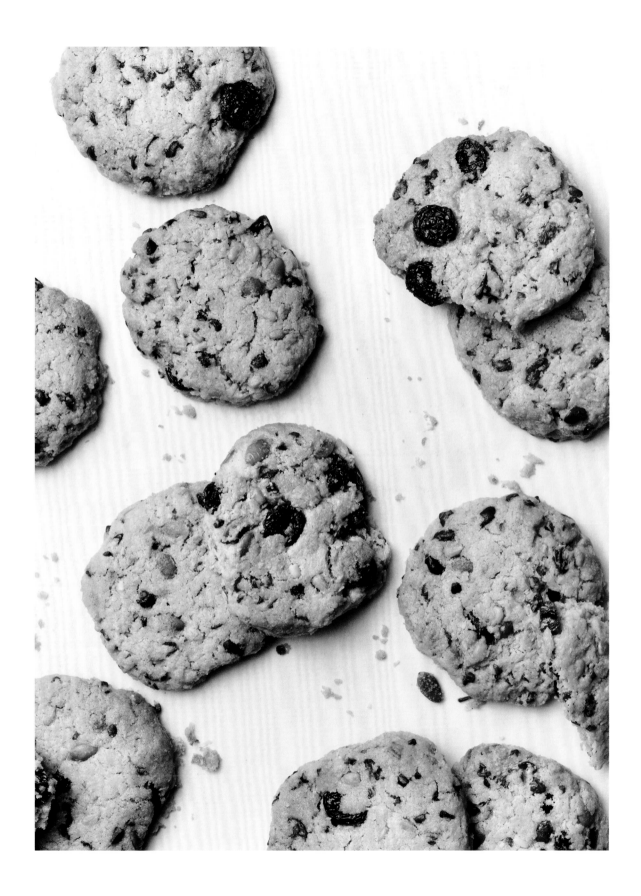

+ **Blood Sugar Balancer**
+ **Colorful** + **Fiber-Rich**
+ **Prebiotic**

2 cups chickpea flour (aka garbanzo bean flour)

3 Tbsp sesame seeds

1 tsp sea salt

½ tsp ground turmeric (optional)

½ tsp garlic powder

⅓ cup extra virgin olive oil

⅓ cup water, plus more as needed

Chickpea Flour Crackers

⊕ **ENERGIZE, FOCUS**

PREP TIME: 20 MINUTES   **COOK TIME:** 20 MINUTES   **MAKES:** 45 CRACKERS

Chickpea flour is such an incredible alternative to regular flour because it's grain-free and naturally gluten-free, but also higher in protein and fiber, which means these crackers will help keep your blood sugar more stable—making them a snack that supports focus and energy. You can enjoy these on their own, or pair with one of our dips, such as Olive Tapenade (page 93) or Roasted Root Veggie Hummus (page 90).

1 Preheat the oven to 350°F.

2 Combine the chickpea flour, sesame seeds, salt, turmeric, and garlic powder in a large bowl.

3 Pour in the oil and water, and stir the mixture together. Use your hands to form the mixture into a ball. The dough should stick together well, but if it's a little dry or flaky, add 1 tsp of water at a time.

4 Place the dough on top of a piece of parchment paper. Place a second sheet of parchment paper overtop, then use a rolling pin to roll out the dough so it's about ⅛-inch thick.

5 Slide the bottom piece of parchment paper, with the dough on it, onto a baking sheet. Remove the top piece of parchment. Cut the dough into 1- × 1-inch squares.

6 Bake for 18–20 minutes, until the crackers are crisp. Keep an eye on them to make sure they don't burn. Remove from the oven and allow the crackers to cool slightly before enjoying. Don't skip the cooling time, as the crackers will crisp up as they dry (they might feel a little soft when you first remove them from the oven). Store in an airtight container for up to 5 days.

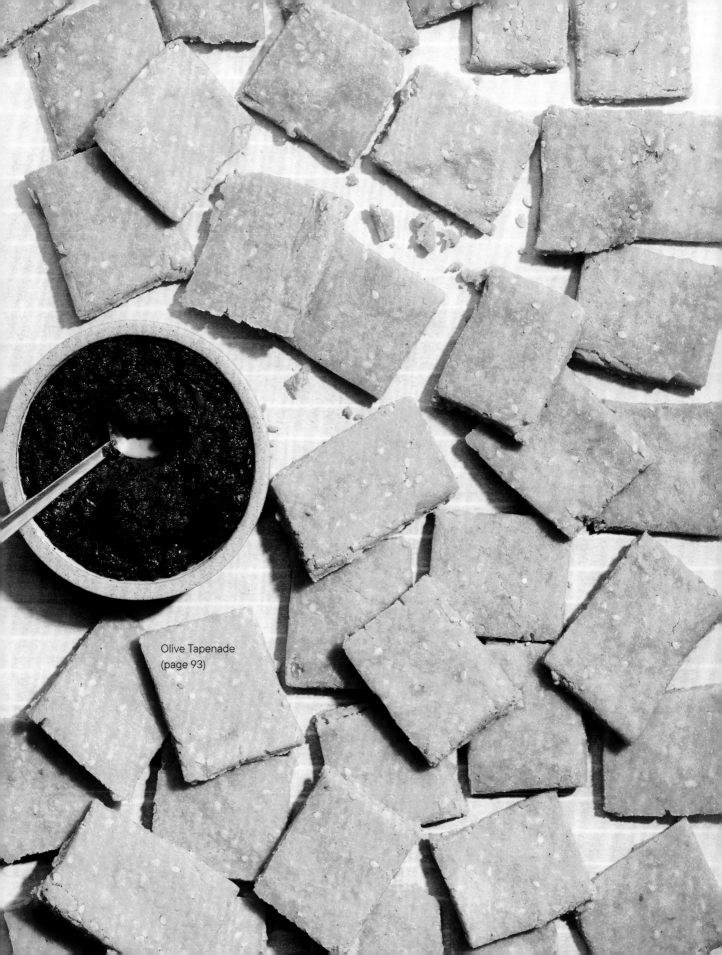

Olive Tapenade
(page 93)

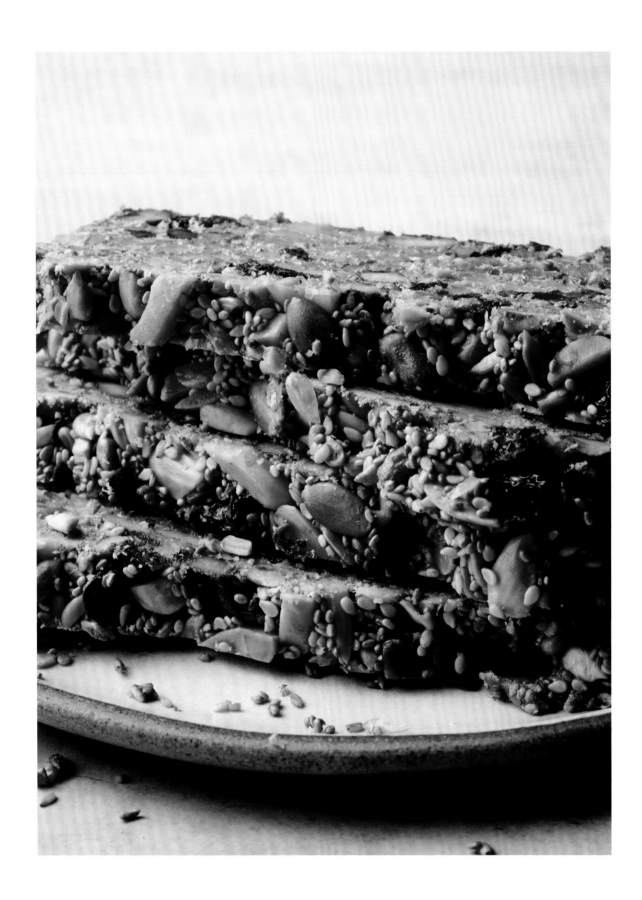

4 eggs

1 cup raw slivered almonds

1 cup raw pistachios or walnuts

1 cup raw pumpkin seeds

1 cup raw sunflower seeds

½ cup sesame seeds

½ cup chia seeds

½ cup roughly chopped dried cranberries

2 tsp sea salt

¼ cup extra virgin olive oil

OPTIONAL TOPPINGS

Butter

Hummus

Yogurt

Sliced avocado

Boiled, scrambled, or over-easy eggs

Hearty Nordic Loaf

⊕ **ENERGIZE, FOCUS**

PREP TIME: 10 MINUTES **COOK TIME:** 50–55 MINUTES

MAKES: ONE 10- × 5-INCH LOAF

Nordic bread, also known as Stone Age bread, originates from Norway, Sweden, and Denmark. This hearty, dense loaf is a combination of nuts, seeds, and eggs, making it protein-rich and a bread that will keep blood sugar steady, so you feel energized and perfectly full after eating it. This a great option for those who don't eat breads with traditional flours or are gluten-free. We like to toast a slice of this bread until it's quite crisp and then slather it with butter.

1 Preheat the oven to 325°F and line a 10- × 5-inch loaf pan with parchment paper.

2 Whisk the eggs in a large bowl, then add the almonds, pistachios, pumpkin seeds, sunflower seeds, sesame seeds, chia seeds, dried cranberries, salt, and oil (leave the nuts and seeds whole).

3 Pour the mixture into the prepared pan and even it out with your hands. Bake for 50–55 minutes, until it's firm to the touch. Remove from the oven and allow to cool before taking out of the pan and slicing.

4 To serve, toast well and top with butter, hummus, yogurt, avocado, eggs, whatever your heart desires. To store, cut the loaf into slices, and keep them in an airtight bag or container in the fridge for up to 1 week or in the freezer for up to 3 months.

Seedy Spelt Loaf

⊕ CALM, UPLIFT

PREP TIME: 10 MINUTES **COOK TIME:** 30–35 MINUTES
MAKES: ONE 10- × 5-INCH LOAF

2 cups light spelt flour

½ cup rye flour

1 tsp baking soda

1 Tbsp baking powder

1 Tbsp + 1 tsp sesame seeds, divided

1 Tbsp + 1 tsp poppy seeds, divided

1 Tbsp + 1 tsp flaxseeds, divided

1 Tbsp + 1 tsp chia seeds, divided

1½ tsp sea salt

1¾ cup plain, unsweetened yogurt or dairy-free yogurt

2 Tbsp runny honey

OPTIONAL TOPPINGS

Butter

Nut/seed butter

Jam

Hummus

Labneh

Sliced avocado

Hard-boiled eggs

If you're a bread-making novice, this is a great loaf to start with. Both spelt and rye, although not gluten-free, have a good amount of fiber that your gut microbes will feast on, improving overall gut health, reducing gut inflammation, and helping create feelings of pleasure, joy, and calm. The yogurt adds a fluffy and light texture, as well as protein. The seeds, especially poppy seeds, elevate this bread by adding a subtle crunch and delicate flavor.

1   Preheat the oven to 400°F and line a 10- × 5-inch loaf pan with parchment paper.

2   In a large bowl, combine the spelt flour, rye flour, baking soda, baking powder, 1 Tbsp sesame seeds, 1 Tbsp poppy seeds, 1 Tbsp flaxseeds, 1 Tbsp chia seeds, and salt. Stir in the yogurt and honey and mix until a batter forms.

3   Pour the dough into the prepared pan. Shake and tap the pan on the counter to even out the batter. Top with the remaining 1 tsp sesame seeds, 1 tsp poppy seeds, 1 tsp flaxseeds, and 1 tsp chia seeds. Bake for 30–35 minutes, until a toothpick inserted into the center comes out clean.

4   Take out of the oven and allow to cool before removing from the pan. Slice and top with butter, nut or seed butter of choice, jam, hummus, labneh, avocado, or hard-boiled eggs.

5   Slice bread and store in the freezer in an airtight bag for up to 2 months. Toast when ready to eat.

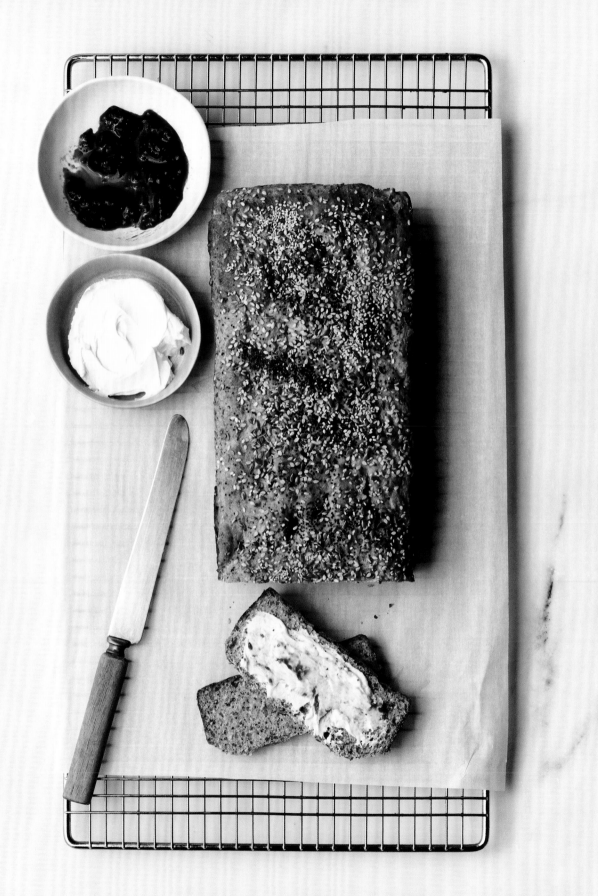

Snickle Snackle Board

⊕ ENERGIZE, FOCUS, UPLIFT

PREP TIME: 10–30 MINUTES **SERVES:** 2–6

FRUIT OPTIONS

Strawberries	Orange slices
Raspberries	Cherries
Blackberries	Grapes
Blueberries	Olives
Apple slices	Cherry tomatoes

VEG OPTIONS

Bell peppers	Fennel
Cucumbers	Celery
Carrots	Radishes

PROTEIN OPTIONS

Nuts and/or seeds of choice

Hard-boiled eggs

Cheese of choice

Meat of choice

DIP OPTIONS

Guacamole

Roasted Red Pepper Walnut
Relish (page 87)

Beet Tahini Yogurt Dip (page 88)

Macadamia Parsley Pesto (page 89)

Roasted Root Veggie Hummus
(page 90)

Olive Tapenade (page 93)

CRACKERS OR BREAD OPTIONS

Sourdough bread slices

Store-bought crackers

Chickpea Flour Crackers (page 106)

Easy Seedy Flax Crackers (page 96)

Hearty Nordic Loaf, toasted
(page 109)

Seedy Spelt Loaf (page 110)

When blood sugar is getting low or children are demanding after-school snacks, our go-to is the snickle snackle board. It's got a variety of textures, flavors, and foods to accommodate cravings and satiate the body. Like any snack board, you can adjust it based on what's in your fridge or what season we happen to be in. This board is filled with a minimum of two kinds of fruits, two kinds of veg, one dip, one variety of bread or crackers, a handful of nuts or seeds, and cheese, or eggs or meat. You could actually use any of the snacks from this chapter to fill your board.

1   Arrange 2 choices each of the fruit and vegetables in small piles on a large serving board, cutting board or platter.

2   Add the 2 proteins you like to the board, placing them where there is an open space next to the fruit and vegetables.

3   Pour 1 or 2 dips into small bowls and place those on the board. If you run out of space, you can serve the bowls on the side.

4   Nestle 1 or 2 of the crackers and bread among the fruit and vegetables.

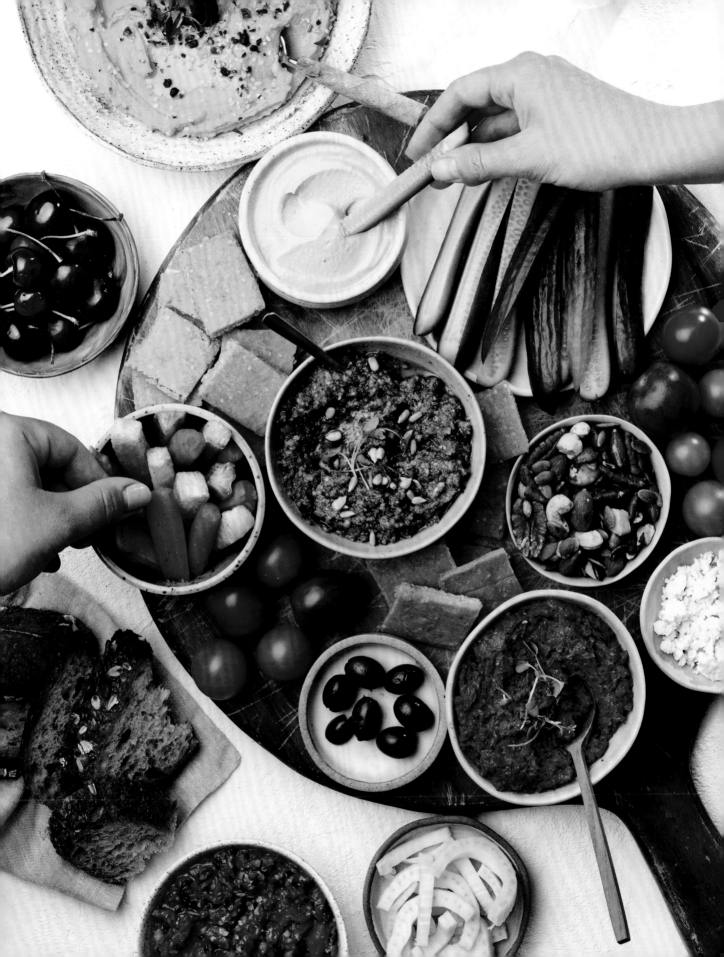

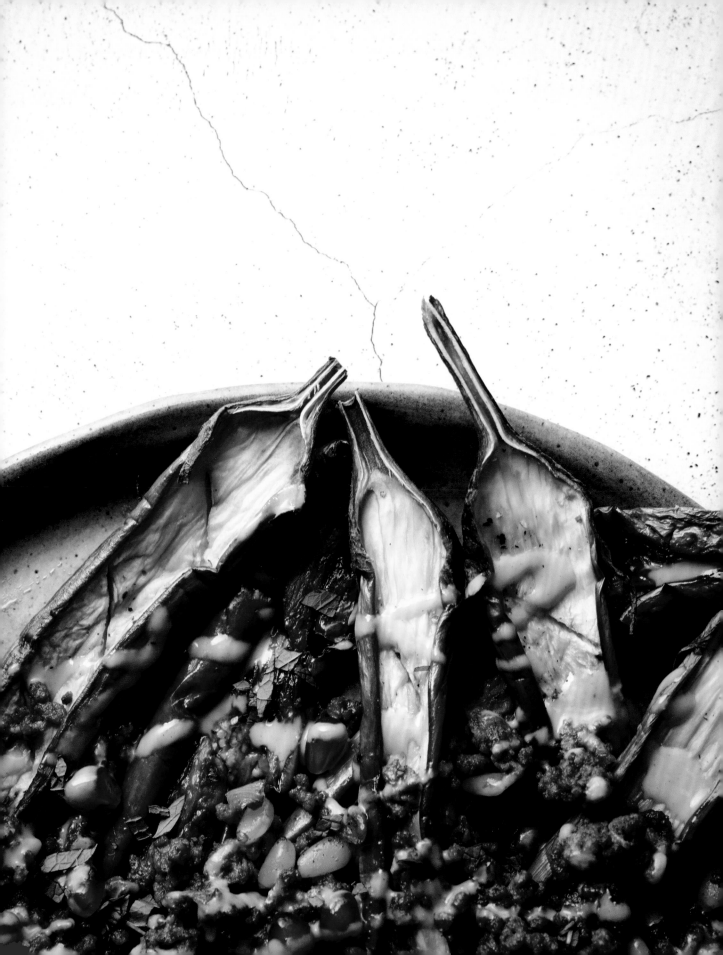

mains

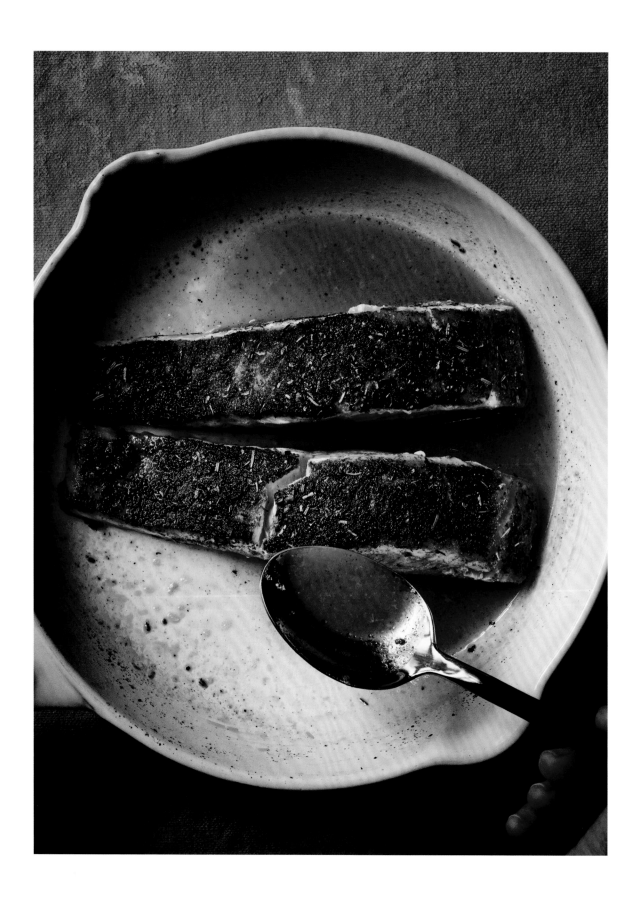

1 Tbsp paprika

2 tsp dried Italian herbs

1 tsp garlic powder

½ tsp sea salt

2 filets of salmon (5 oz each)

1 Tbsp extra virgin olive oil

½ cup freshly squeezed orange
   juice (from 1–2 oranges)

1 Tbsp orange zest, for garnish

¼ cup roughly chopped fresh
   cilantro or parsley, for
   garnish

Orange-Infused Blackened Salmon

⊕ ENERGIZE, FOCUS, UPLIFT

PREP TIME: 3 MINUTES   **COOK TIME:** 15 MINUTES   **SERVES:** 2

We often end up roasting salmon in the oven—it's a quick and easy way to prepare it but, let's face it, simple oven-baked salmon can get boring. Searing salmon is so much more interesting, and thanks to this spice rub, the salmon becomes even more flavorful and crispy as it browns. Fresh orange juice brings the perfect amount of sweetness and keeps the fish nice and tender. Of all the fish out there, salmon has one of the highest amounts of omega-3 per serving, plus you'll get vitamins D and B_6 to support your mood—these are all vital nutrients to prevent and ease depression and anxiety. We love serving this salmon with roasted vegetables, such as our Crispy Smashed Potatoes with Yogurt Sauce (page 184) or Roasted Jerusalem Artichokes, Beets, and Cauliflower with Pistachio Dukkah (page 177).

1   Mix together the paprika, Italian herbs, garlic powder, and salt on a large plate, then spread the spice rub out evenly across the surface of the plate.

2   Pat the salmon dry with paper towel. Place the salmon flesh side down in the spice rub to coat it. Set aside on another plate and repeat with the remaining piece of salmon.

3   Heat the oil in a large skillet over medium heat, swirling it around to coat the bottom. Once the oil is hot, place the salmon, flesh side down, in the pan.

4   After about 3–5 minutes, the spices will start to brown as the fish cooks. Pour in the orange juice and continue to cook until most of the liquid has evaporated and caramelized. Flip the fish over and cook for another 5–7 minutes. The spices will look blackened, and if you gently puncture the salmon with a fork, it should flake easily. If the fish is very thick, place it in a preheated 350°F oven for a few minutes to complete cooking, to an internal temperature of 145°F.

5   Garnish with the orange zest and cilantro just before serving.

1 lb trout fillet

½ tsp sea salt, plus a pinch

Pinch of pepper

2 eggs

2 Tbsp mayonnaise

1 Tbsp Dijon mustard

2 Tbsp finely chopped fresh parsley

2 Tbsp finely chopped fresh dill

3 Tbsp finely chopped chives

¼ cup almond flour or 2 Tbsp oat flour

½ tsp granulated garlic powder

½ cup Yogurt Sauce (page 184)

Green Herb Trout Burgers

⊕ ENERGIZE, FOCUS, UPLIFT

PREP TIME: 15 MINUTES **COOK TIME:** 35 MINUTES
MAKES: 9 SMALL BURGERS

We love salmon, but know that it often becomes the go-to fish for so many of us, even when there really are so many other fish in the sea! Trout is a great replacement for salmon in fish burgers because it's mild and also a good source of omega-3, the nourishing fat that protects the brain and helps us feel happier. This high-protein recipe freezes well, so make a double batch for easy, quick meals in the future! We often like to eat these burgers for lunch, especially paired with leftover roasted vegetables—try it with Our Favorite Roasted Veggie Medley (page 183)—or a salad.

1 Preheat the oven to 375°F and line 2 baking sheets with parchment paper.

2 Place the trout on one of the prepared baking sheets and season it with a pinch of salt and pepper. Bake for 15 minutes or until the fish is cooked through and flakes easily with a fork. Once the fish is cooked, remove it from the oven, keeping the oven on, and let cool for 5–10 minutes.

3 Whisk together the eggs, mayonnaise, and mustard in a large bowl. Add the parsley, dill, chives, almond flour, garlic powder, and ½ tsp salt. Flake the cooled fish into the bowl, removing the skin (the fish will flake easily with a fork into small pieces). Mix everything together to combine evenly.

4 Use your hands or a ¼-cup measuring cup to scoop and shape the mixture into 9 small ½-inch thick burgers. Place them on the second prepared baking sheet. Bake for 15 minutes, then flip and cook for an additional 5 minutes, until lightly golden.

5 You can eat these trout burgers with a bun, on top of a salad, or with roasted vegetables. We love to dollop the yogurt sauce on top each burger for an extra boost of flavor and probiotics. Leftovers can be stored in the fridge for up to 3 days or in the freezer for up to 2 months.

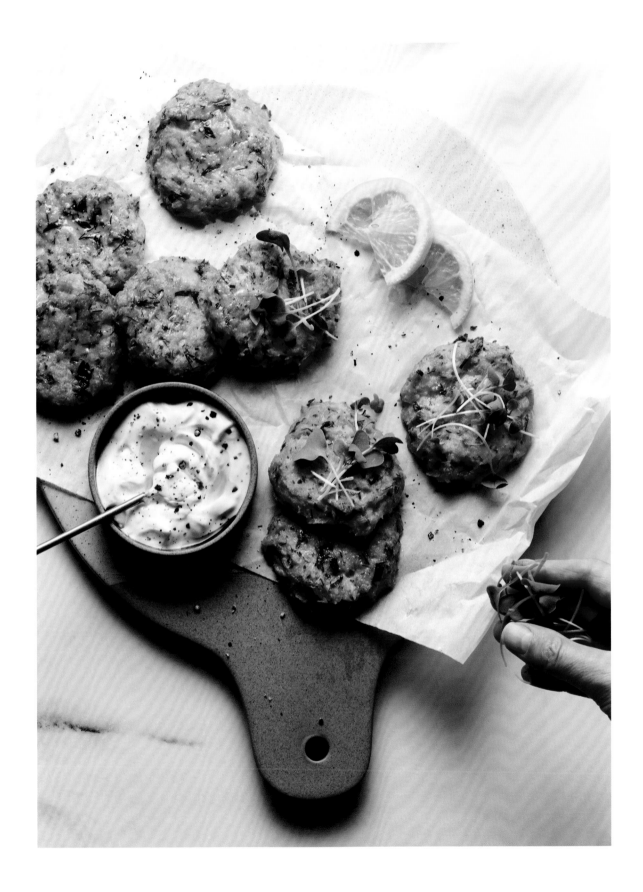

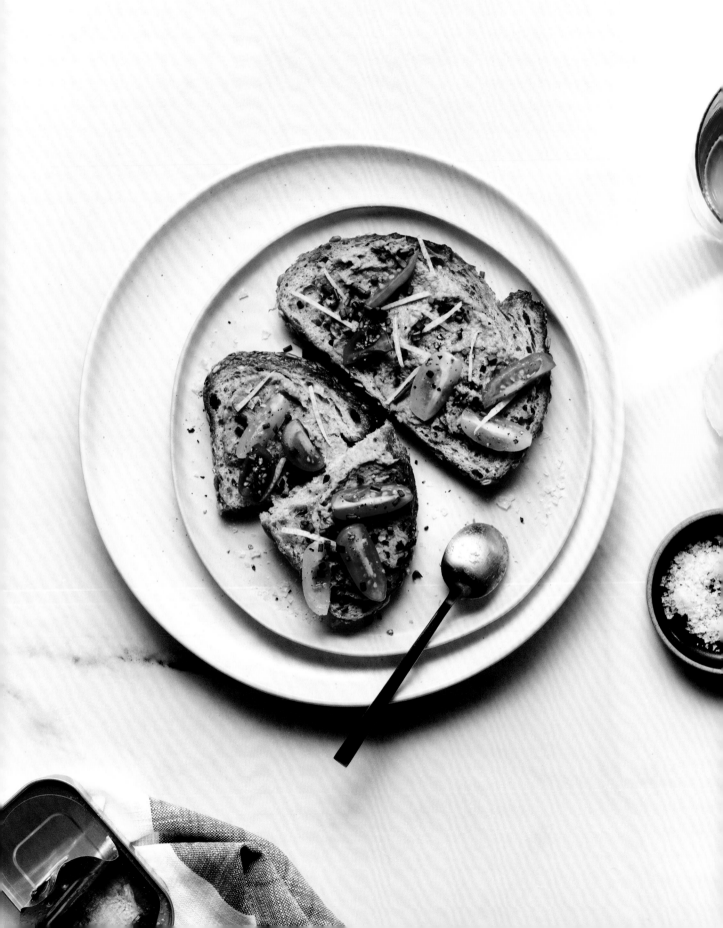

Sardine Pâté with Sourdough Toasties

⊕ ENERGIZE, FOCUS, UPLIFT

PREP TIME: 5 MINUTES **SERVES:** 4

+ Blood Sugar Balancer

+ Healthy Fats

+ Protein-Powered

1 tin of sardines, packed in extra virgin olive oil (look for BPA-free packaging)

2 Tbsp freshly squeezed lemon juice

1 Tbsp butter, at room temperature

1 tsp Dijon mustard

Sea salt and pepper to taste

4 slices sourdough bread

Handful of chives (or other fresh herbs you like), chopped, for garnish

Fresh lemon zest, for garnish (optional)

7 cherry tomatoes, halved, for garnish (optional)

We've always wanted to love sardines but, like so many people, we were apprehensive about eating them. Eating a whole (though tiny) fish might not seem super appealing, but sardines are one of the best food sources of omega-3, which you'll want to eat more of to help reduce anxiety and depression. When blended up into a pâté, you'll find that the creamy, rich texture pairs wonderfully with crispy sourdough (or crackers). This recipe is perfect for lunch—since it's high in protein, it will keep you fueled and focused after eating. Try it with a salad, such as our Pretty in Purple Salad (page 176).

1 Place the sardines, 1 Tbsp of oil from the can, lemon juice, butter, and mustard in a food processor (or mini blender) and blend until you have a smooth, creamy mixture. Season with salt and pepper.

2 Toast the bread. We prefer the toast crunchy—almost crisp—to complement the smooth texture of the pâté.

3 Spread the pâté on the toast and garnish with the chives, lemon zest, and tomatoes. Store extra pâté in an airtight container in the fridge for up to 3 days.

One-Pan Miso Braised Cod and Leeks

⊕ ENERGIZE, FOCUS, UPLIFT

PREP TIME: 10 MINUTES **COOK TIME:** 22 MINUTES **SERVES:** 2

3 leeks

2 Tbsp extra virgin olive oil

½ tsp coconut sugar

¼ tsp sea salt

A few cracks of pepper

2 cod fillets (5 oz each)

½ cup chicken broth or vegetable broth

½ lemon, zested and juiced

1 Tbsp white miso paste

¼ cup chopped pistachios

1 green onion, sliced, for garnish (optional)

Leeks are one of the best prebiotic foods to help feed the beneficial microbes in your gut. When they're braised, they become soft and sweet. In this dish, they also caramelize from the coconut sugar. Miso and fish are a match made in heaven, not only for your taste buds but for your whole body—miso contains ferments that increase the good bacteria in your gut (they make the feel-good neurotransmitters that help you feel more positive), and cod is rich in B_{12} and omega-3, both nutrients that can help ease depression. Serve this dish with quinoa or rice, or with our Coconut Milk Cauliflower Rice (page 181) or Golden Miso "Risotto" (page 180).

1   Trim the root of the leek and cut off any darker leaves at the top— you'll be using mostly the white part. Slice the leeks in half length- wise and rinse them well. If the leeks are particularly gritty, soak them in a large bowl of water for 7–10 minutes, and then rinse again.

2   Place a large, wide skillet over medium heat, add the oil, and swirl it around to coat the bottom. Sprinkle in the coconut sugar, ⅛ tsp salt, and pepper, stirring to mix. Place the leeks cut side down in the oil mixture. (If the leeks are too long for the pan, cut them smaller to fit). Cook for 3 minutes, then flip and cook for another 2–4 minutes, until slightly caramelized.

3   Season the cod with remaining salt and pepper and place on top of the leeks.

4   In a small bowl, whisk together the broth, lemon juice, and miso. Pour the mixture over the cod, allowing it to drip on the leeks below. Cover the skillet, turn the heat to low, and simmer for 10–15 minutes, until the fish is cooked through and leeks are buttery and soft.

5   Remove from the heat, sprinkle with the lemon zest, pistachios, and green onion. Season with sea salt and pepper, if needed.

NOTE: *Save the green top part of the leeks for homemade soups or stocks. Or slice them thinly and sauté with butter, minced garlic, and a pinch each of sea salt and pepper for a simple side.*

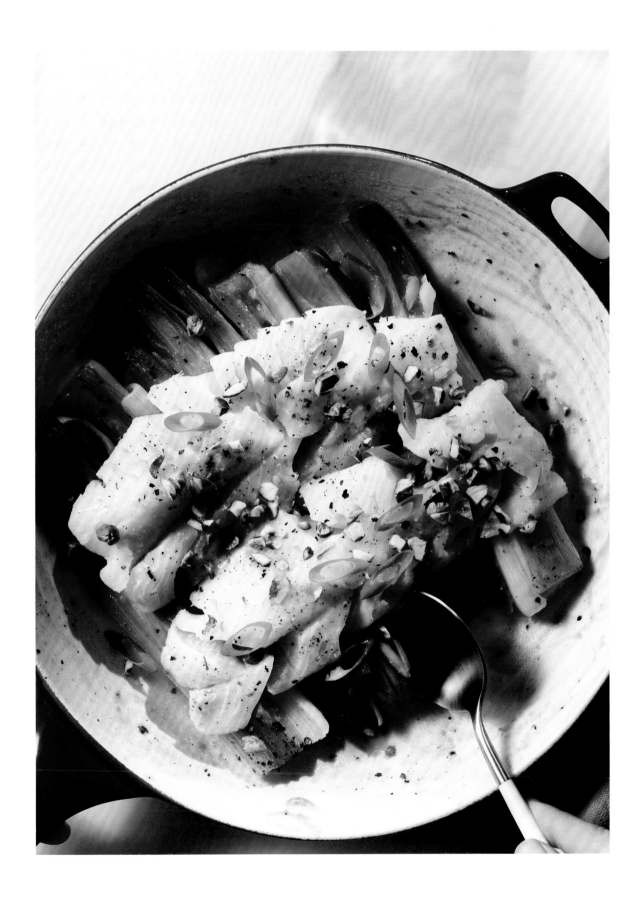

ROASTED CABBAGE WEDGES

2 Tbsp + 2 tsp extra virgin olive oil, divided

1 small green or purple cabbage

½ tsp sea salt, divided

A few cracks of pepper

ZHOUG SALMON

¼ cup extra virgin olive oil, plus more for drizzling

2 Tbsp freshly squeezed lemon juice

2 Tbsp water, plus more as needed

1 bunch cilantro, including stems (about 2 cups)

1 small garlic clove

½ tsp ground cumin

¼ tsp ground cardamom

¼ tsp sea salt, plus more for seasoning

A few cracks of pepper, plus more for seasoning

4 salmon fillets (4–6 oz each)

Sheet-Pan Zhoug Salmon with Roasted Cabbage Wedges

⊕ **ENERGIZE, FOCUS, UPLIFT**

PREP TIME: 10 MINUTES   **COOK TIME:** 35 MINUTES   **SERVES:** 4

Zhoug is a spicy cilantro sauce originating from Yemen. This version is milder than traditional preparations, but the flavors are still bright and zippy. Who doesn't love a good sheet-pan dinner with minimal dishes and prep? When you roast cabbage, it becomes softer, slightly crispy, and sweet. Plus, it's one of those vegetables that can last in your fridge for a while, so it's easy to keep on hand.

1   Preheat the oven to 375°F.

Make the Cabbage

2   Drizzle the bottom of a baking sheet with 2 Tbsp of oil, and place it in the oven.

3   Slice the cabbage into 8 wedges. You may only need to use one half of the cabbage if it's very large. Remove the hot baking sheet from the oven and place the cabbage on it—you'll hear sizzles. Drizzle the remaining 2 tsp oil overtop the cabbage, and season with salt and pepper. Roast for 15 minutes.

Prepare the Zhoug Salmon

4   Place the oil, lemon juice, water, cilantro, garlic, cumin, cardamom, ¼ tsp salt, and pepper in a food processor or blender. Blitz until vibrant green and a similar consistency to pesto.

5   Once the cabbage has roasted for 15 minutes, remove from the oven, flip the wedges, and move them to the outer sides of the baking sheet to make room for the salmon. Place the salmon in the middle of the baking sheet, drizzle with a little oil, and season with the salt and pepper.

6   Roast the salmon and cabbage for 15–20 minutes, until the fish is 145°F. Fish is perfectly cooked when the thickest section gently flakes when punctured with a fork. Once the fish is cooked, remove from the oven and generously spoon the zhoug over the fish and cabbage.

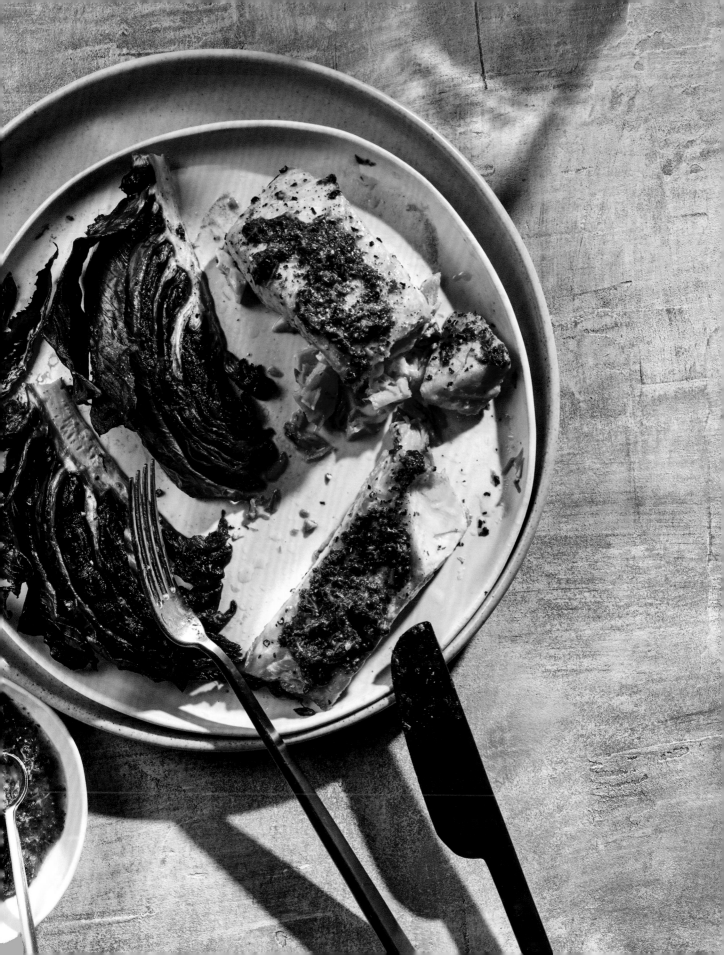

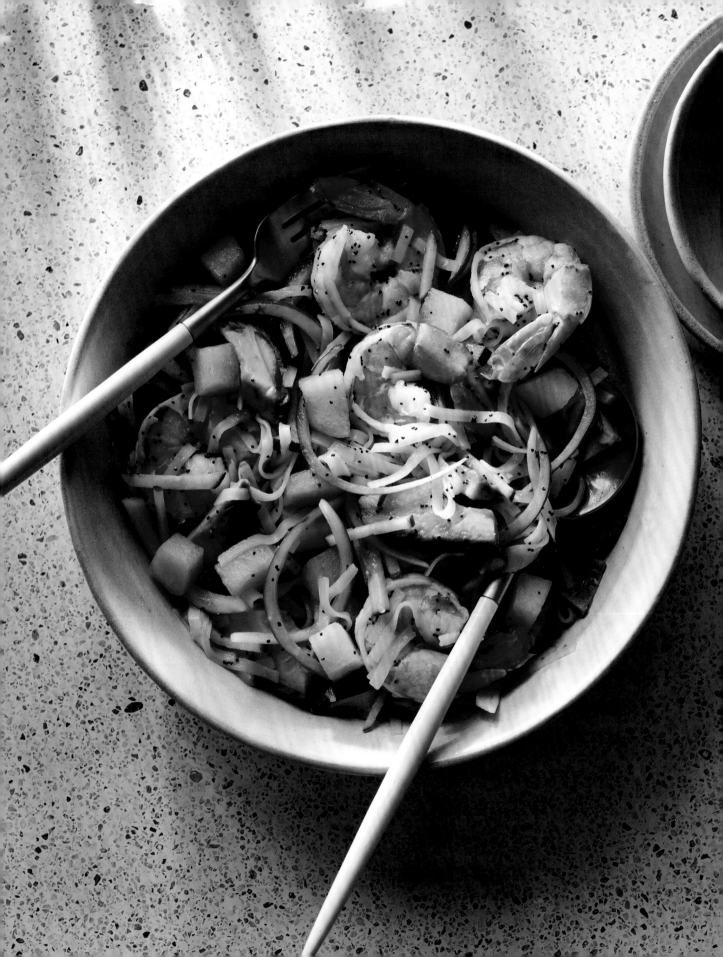

Melon Poppy Seed Shrimp Salad

➕ **ENERGIZE, FOCUS, UPLIFT**
PREP TIME: 25 MINUTES   COOK TIME: 10 MINUTES   SERVES: 4

+ **Blood Sugar Balancer**
+ **Colorful + Fiber-Rich**
+ **Healthy Fats + Prebiotic**
+ **Protein-Powered**

1 lime, halved

½ tsp sea salt

8 black peppercorns

1 lb large, raw shrimp, peeled and deveined (tails can be left on, if you prefer)

½ package of thin rice noodles (optional)

2 radishes, cut in matchsticks or half-moons

⅓ cucumber, cut in matchsticks or half-moons

1 cup chopped snap peas or snow peas

½ cup cantaloupe, cut in ½-inch cubes

¼ small red onion, thinly sliced, or ¼ cup pickled red onion

½ –1 avocado, peeled, pitted, and sliced

½ –1 cup roughly torn mixed fresh herbs (mint, basil, and/ or cilantro)

1 Tbsp poppy seeds

HONEY LIME VINAIGRETTE

⅓ cup extra virgin olive oil

⅓ cup lime juice

¼ cup + 1 Tbsp rice vinegar

1 Tbsp honey

1 small garlic clove, minced

½ tsp sea salt

A few cracks of pepper

Fresh and colorful, this salad is a one-bowl meal with all the vegetables, protein, and healthy fat you need for balanced blood sugar, to feel full, focused, and energized. The sweet-and-sour dressing brings everything together in this summery, uplifting meal that was inspired by our friend Sonia Wong, of the blog *saltnpepperhere*. We love the beautiful array of colors here, pastel orange and purple and our favorite, green—you can be sure that you're eating a variety of micronutrients and minerals that support you in feeling more joyful.

1 Pour 16 cups of water into a pot, squeeze in the juice of half a lime, and then put both lime halves in the pot, add the salt and pepper-corns, and bring to a boil. Add the shrimp, cover the pot, and remove from the heat. Let stand for 5 minutes or until the shrimp turn pink. Using a slotted spoon, immediately transfer the shrimp to a sieve and run under cold water for 45 seconds to stop the cooking.

2 If you're using rice noodles, boil a pot of water, turn off the heat, and add the noodles, giving them a quick stir. Let sit for 7–10 minutes, then drain and rinse under cold water.

3 To make the vinaigrette, whisk together the oil, lime juice, rice vinegar, honey, garlic, salt, and pepper.

4 In a large bowl, toss together the shrimp, radishes, cucumber, snap peas, cantaloupe, red onion, and noodles. Pour the vinaigrette overtop and toss to coat.

5 Top with avocado, fresh herbs, and poppy seeds. Give it all another gentle toss to incorporate the toppings. It's best to enjoy this recipe right away.

Hemp Mushroom Veggie Burgers with Thyme and Balsamic

⊕ ENERGIZE, FOCUS, UPLIFT

PREP TIME: 10 MINUTES **COOK TIME:** 45–50 MINUTES **MAKES:** 9 BURGERS

2 tsp extra virgin olive oil

2 shallots, sliced

½ tsp dried thyme or 2 tsp fresh thyme leaves

2 large garlic cloves, chopped

8 oz cremini mushrooms, sliced

1½ cups cooked short grain brown rice (see note)

½ cup hemp seeds

1 Tbsp ground flaxseed

1 Tbsp balsamic vinegar

1 Tbsp tamari or coconut aminos

¼ tsp sea salt

Pinch of pepper

NOTE: *To cook the rice, place ¾ cup short grain brown rice, 1½ cups of water, and a dash of sea salt in a pot. Bring to a boil, cover, and simmer on low for 35 minutes or until the water is absorbed.*

We've made so many types of veggie burgers over the years, and this one is unique. Hemp seeds are an amazing source of protein and plant-based omega-3, which help boost brain and neurotransmitter function, so you feel more balanced and at ease. Usually, these seeds are just sprinkled on top of salads, but if you have a bag of them sitting around, why not incorporate them into a delicious recipe? (And if you don't have them on hand, you can use walnuts instead—both walnuts and hemp seeds support brain health.) Enjoy these burgers with our Rainbow Mediterranean Salad (page 165).

1 Heat the oil in a medium stainless steel or cast-iron skillet. Add the shallots and sauté for 2 to 3 minutes, until they begin to soften. Toss in the thyme and garlic, stir, and cook for another minute. Add the mushrooms and give them a nice stir along with the shallots and garlic, then let sit undisturbed for 2 minutes—this will help the moisture from the mushrooms evaporate. Then continue to sauté and stir for 5 minutes or until the mushrooms have reduced in size and browned.

2 Preheat the oven to 375°F and line a baking sheet with parchment paper.

3 Place the mushroom mixture, rice, hemp seeds, ground flaxseed, vinegar, tamari, salt, and pepper in a food processor and pulse a few times, until the ingredients comes together in a sticky mixture. Don't overprocess it into a puree—you want the mixture to have some texture, with small pieces of mushroom and rice remaining.

4 Scoop out the mixture and shape into 9 patties with your hands. Place the patties on the prepared baking sheet. Bake for 20 minutes, then flip and bake for 10–15 minutes more, until the burgers are golden brown and crisp.

5 Store leftover burgers in an airtight container in the fridge for up to 4 days or in the freezer in an airtight container or bag for up to 2 months.

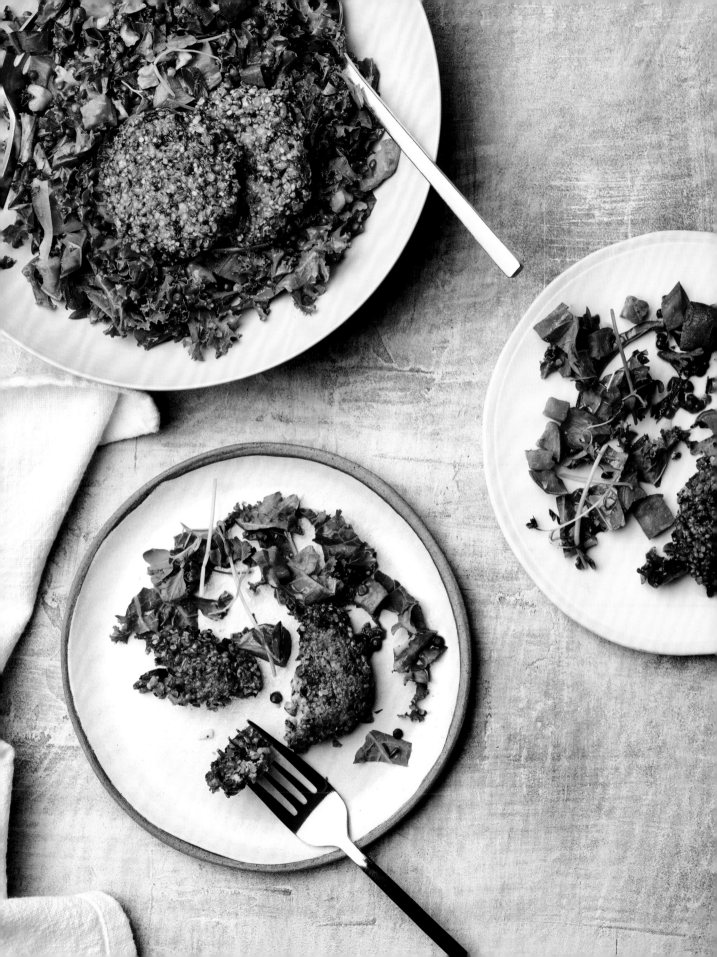

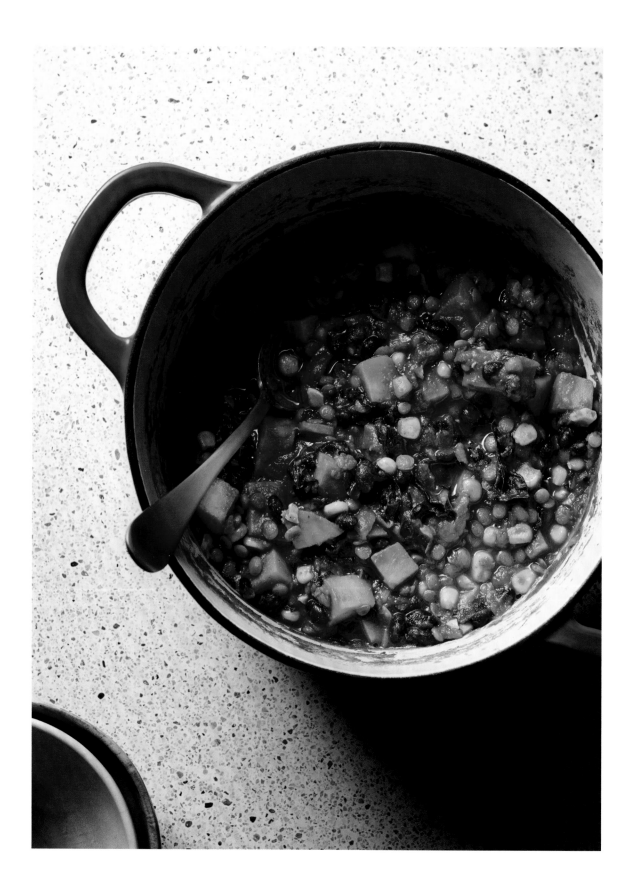

Cozy Lentil and Black Bean Chili

+ Blood Sugar Balancer

+ Fiber-Rich + Prebiotic

+ Protein-Powered

⊕ CALM, ENERGIZE, FOCUS, UPLIFT

PREP TIME: 7 MINUTES **COOK TIME:** 35 MINUTES **SERVES:** 4

1 Tbsp extra virgin olive oil

4 small garlic cloves, minced

1 celery stalk, diced

1 Tbsp chili powder

1 tsp ground cumin

1 tsp paprika

1 tsp onion powder

½ tsp sea salt

A few cracks of pepper

1 sweet potato, cubed

1 can (14 oz) diced tomatoes

1½ cups vegetable broth

⅓ cup dried green lentils, rinsed

1 can (14 oz) black beans

½ cup frozen corn kernels

2 cups chopped green kale

1 lime, cut in 4 wedges, for garnish

1 avocado, peeled, pitted, and sliced, for garnish

¼ cup fresh cilantro leaves, for garnish

When it comes to incorporating a wide array of colorful vegetables into your meals, this recipe is a fantastic one to do just that, especially during the colder months. Remember, eating a variety of produce is linked with feeling better, and it can be easy to do that by throwing together a salad. But when you want a warming, cozy meal, sometimes it can be a little more challenging to get that variety. This dish includes plenty of plant-based protein as well, thanks to the black beans and green lentils. We make this chili with a mild level of spice, but feel free to add more chili powder if you like things spicy!

1   Heat the oil in a large pot set over medium heat. Add the garlic and celery, and sauté for 30 seconds or until the garlic is fragrant. Add the chili powder, cumin, paprika, onion powder, salt, and pepper and sauté for 2–3 minutes.

2   Stir in the sweet potato, tomatoes, broth, and lentils. Turn up the heat to high. When the mixture is about to boil, turn the heat down to low, cover, and simmer for 20 minutes, until the sweet potatoes and lentils are softened.

3   Give the chili a good stir, then add the black beans, corn, and kale. Cover and simmer for another 10 minutes, until the corn and kale are cooked. Taste and add more salt or pepper, if you like.

4   To serve, portion the chili into bowls. Garnish with lime wedges, avocado and cilantro. Chili is the perfect dish for leftovers. Store in an airtight container in the fridge for up to 4 days or in the freezer for up to 3 months.

Herby Lemon Chickpeas and Beets

⊕ CALM, ENERGIZE, FOCUS, UPLIFT

PREP TIME: 10 MINUTES **COOK TIME:** 30–60 MINUTES **SERVES:** 2

1 lb purple and golden beets (about 4 medium or 8 mini)

4 Tbsp extra virgin olive oil, divided

Sea salt and pepper

⅓ cup raw walnuts

1 can (19 oz) chickpeas, drained and rinsed, or 1¾ cups cooked chickpeas

¼ cup chopped fresh parsley, plus more for garnish (optional)

3 Tbsp chopped green onions or chives, plus more for garnish (optional)

2 Tbsp chopped fresh basil, plus more for garnish (optional)

3 Tbsp chopped sun-dried tomatoes

1 Tbsp freshly squeezed lemon juice

1 Tbsp apple cider vinegar

1 garlic clove, minced

3 tsp tamari

½ cup goat feta or dairy-free "feta" cheese (optional)

4 hard-boiled eggs, peeled and quartered (optional)

If you need a quick recipe that keeps well in the fridge for a few days, this one's for you. The vibrant herbs, fresh lemon, and savory sun-dried tomatoes are delicious when paired with earthy beets and crunchy walnuts. It's ideal for lunch, and it's easy to build upon—you can throw in some cooked quinoa if you need more carbs or add leftover cooked chicken for more protein. Beets and chickpeas are a double win for your gut—lots of fiber and prebiotic resistant starch to feed the good bacteria, so they can get to work making you feel more cheerful. Chickpeas and beets also offer B vitamins, for your neurotransmitter production, which helps ease stress.

1   Preheat the oven to 400°F.

2   Trim the beets to remove any stringy or tough parts. Place them in a small baking dish and rub with 2 Tbsp oil and salt and pepper to taste. Cover the baking dish with aluminum foil or a small sheet pan. Roast for about 30 minutes for mini beets or for about 60 minutes for medium beets, until tender.

3   While the beets are roasting, spread the walnuts on a small baking sheet and roast in the 400°F oven for 5–7 minutes, until lightly browned.

4   Remove the beets from the oven and, once they are cool enough to handle, remove the skin. Cut the beets into wedges or thin rounds.

5   Toss together the chickpeas, parsley, green onions, basil, and sun-dried tomatoes in a large bowl. Add the lemon juice, vinegar, garlic, and tamari. You can adjust the seasoning as needed—you might want extra lemon juice or more green onions.

6   Add the beets and toss to mix. Top with the roasted walnuts. If you're using feta cheese, sprinkle it overtop, and top it all with hard-boiled eggs, if you like. Feel free to sprinkle with more chopped fresh herbs before serving.

7   Store leftovers in an airtight container in the fridge for up to 4 days.

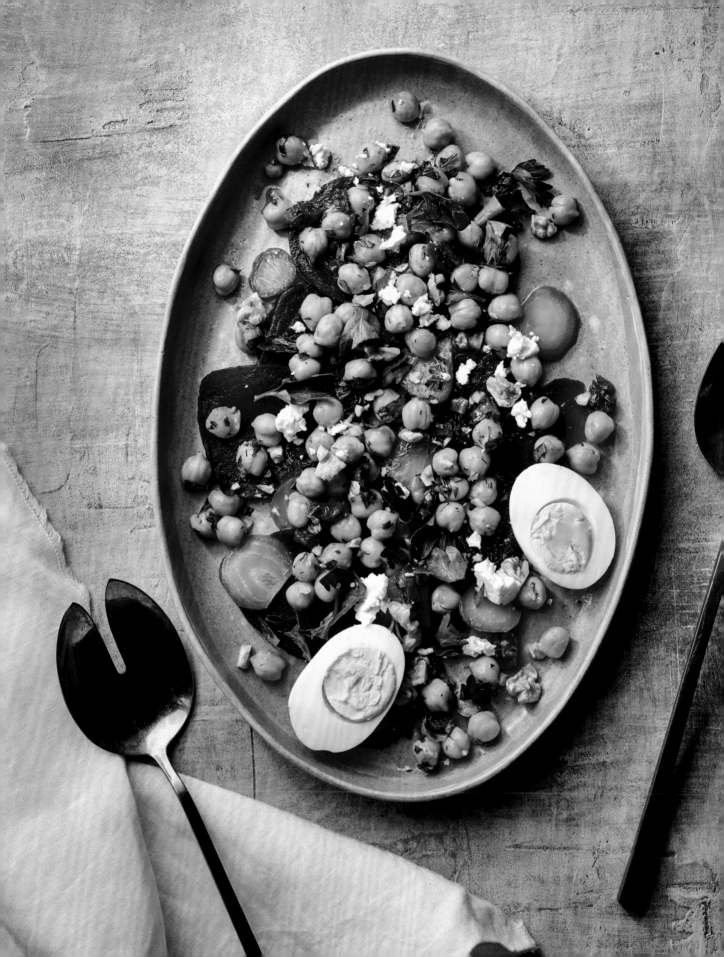

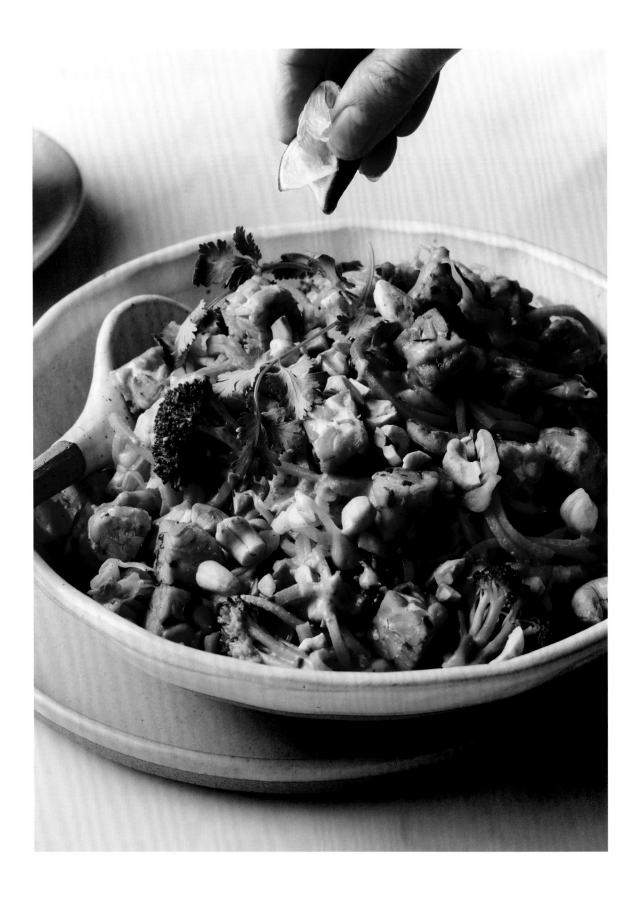

ALMOND SAUCE

⅓ cup tamari

¼ cup freshly squeezed lime juice (about 1½ limes)

⅓ cup natural almond butter

1½ Tbsp maple syrup

1 small garlic clove, minced

¼ to ⅓ cup water

SWEET POTATO NOODLES AND TEMPEH

1–3 Tbsp extra virgin olive oil, divided

3 garlic cloves, sliced

1 head broccoli, cut in florets

1½ lb sweet potato (about 2 medium), spiralized, or store-bought spiralized sweet potato noodles

3 cups shredded green cabbage

1 (8 oz) block tempeh, cubed

1 lime, cut in 4 wedges

¼ cup chopped cilantro, for garnish

⅓ cup roasted cashews, for garnish

Sweet Potato Noodles with Almond Sauce and Tempeh

⊕ **CALM, ENERGIZE, FOCUS, UPLIFT**

PREP TIME: 15 MINUTES **COOK TIME:** 20 MINUTES **SERVES:** 4

Sarah: Many years ago, I went on a women's retreat and fell in love with a sweet potato noodle dish they served, a recipe by Rachel Molenda. This dish is inspired by that. Sweet potatoes provide vitamins, phytonutrients, and fiber to support your gut and neurotransmitters to help you feel balanced, focused, and joyful. You'll love this creamy and tangy almond butter sauce—it works on any vegetable, so sub in whatever you have.

Make the Almond Sauce

1 Place the tamari, lime juice, almond butter, maple syrup, garlic, and water in a blender (you can add water as desired). Blend until you have a smooth sauce. Set aside.

Make the Sweet Potato Noodles and Tempeh

2 Heat 1 Tbsp of oil in a large skillet set over medium-high heat. Once hot, add the garlic and cook for 30 seconds or until fragrant. Add the broccoli and sauté for 2–3 minutes; it will turn bright green. Toss in the sweet potato noodles and stir-fry for 5–7 minutes, until they begin to soften. If the pan is getting dry, add an additional 1 Tbsp of oil. Add the cabbage and cook for 5 minutes, stirring occasionally. Once the veggies are tender, transfer to a large bowl and set aside.

3 Place the skillet back on the heat. Heat the remaining 1 Tbsp oil over medium-high heat and sear the tempeh on one side for about 4 minutes, until crisp, then flip and sear on the second side for about 3 minutes, until crisp.

4 Transfer the tempeh to the bowl with the veggies and toss together. Gradually add the sauce.

5 Garnish with the cilantro and cashews, and serve each portion with a lime wedge.

CRISPY CHICKPEAS AND CAULIFLOWER

1 can (19 oz) chickpeas, drained and rinsed, or 1¾ cups cooked chickpeas

1 small cauliflower, cut in small florets (about 4 cups)

2 Tbsp extra virgin olive oil

¾ tsp garlic powder

¾ tsp sumac

2 tsp balsamic vinegar

½ tsp sea salt

Pinch of pepper

LEMONY TAHINI YOGURT

½ cup plain Greek yogurt or dairy-free yogurt

1 Tbsp freshly squeezed lemon juice

1 Tbsp tahini

¼ tsp sumac

¼ tsp sea salt

Pinch of pepper

TO SERVE

Squeeze of lemon

Drizzle of extra virgin olive oil

Handful of fresh cilantro or parsley, chopped

Crispy Chickpeas and Cauliflower over Lemony Tahini Yogurt

⊕ **CALM, ENERGIZE, FOCUS, UPLIFT**

PREP TIME: 15 MINUTES **COOK TIME:** 25–30 MINUTES **SERVES:** 2

Chickpeas are high in protein and B vitamins, which help support healthy neurotransmitters and a good mood. We love the yogurt here because it's an easy way to incorporate probiotics into a savory meal, so they can strengthen your gut to keep you feeling healthy and uplifted. This recipe pairs well with our Creamy Squash Miso Soup (page 173).

1 Preheat the oven to 400°F and line a baking sheet with parchment paper.

Roast the Chickpeas and Cauliflower

2 Place the chickpeas and cauliflower on the baking sheet and toss together with the oil, garlic powder, sumac, vinegar, salt, and pepper. Mix everything to evenly coat the chickpeas and cauliflower. Spread the chickpeas and cauliflower evenly on the sheet, so everything can get crisp.

3 Roast for 25–30 minutes. Remove from the oven and give everything a good stir. The chickpeas should be crisp, and the cauliflower will be getting crisp and golden. If the cauliflower isn't browned enough, put it back in the oven for another 5 minutes.

Make the Lemony Tahini Yogurt

4 In a small bowl, stir together the yogurt, lemon juice, tahini, sumac, salt, and pepper. Spread the lemony tahini yogurt on a serving platter or large plate.

5 Place the roasted chickpeas and cauliflower on top of the lemony tahini yogurt. Finish with a squeeze of lemon, a drizzle of oil, and a sprinkle of cilantro.

6 If you're not eating right away or want to save leftovers, spread only the portions of chickpeas and cauliflower to be eaten over a small scoop of the lemony tahini yogurt. Store the leftover sauce and the chickpea mixture in separate airtight containers in the fridge for up to 4 days.

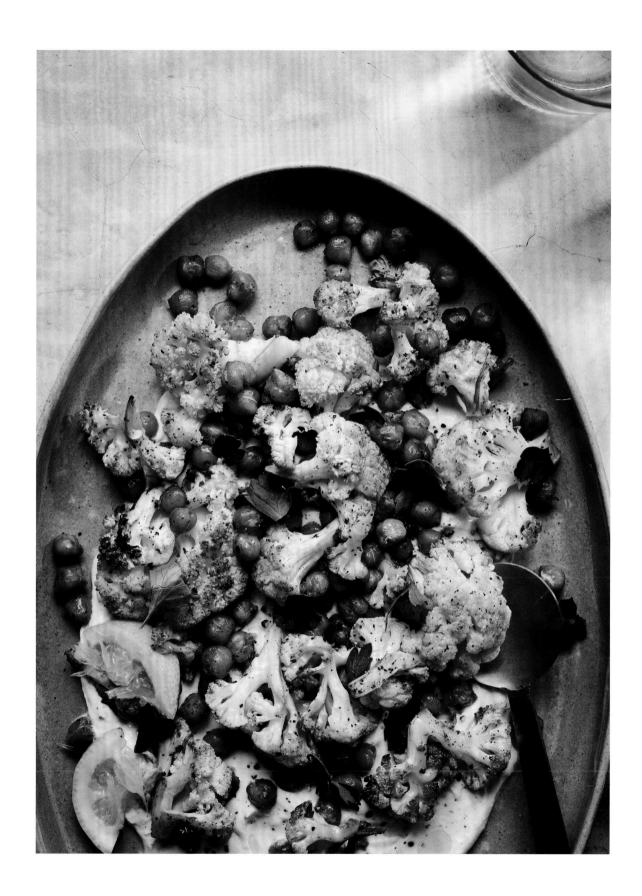

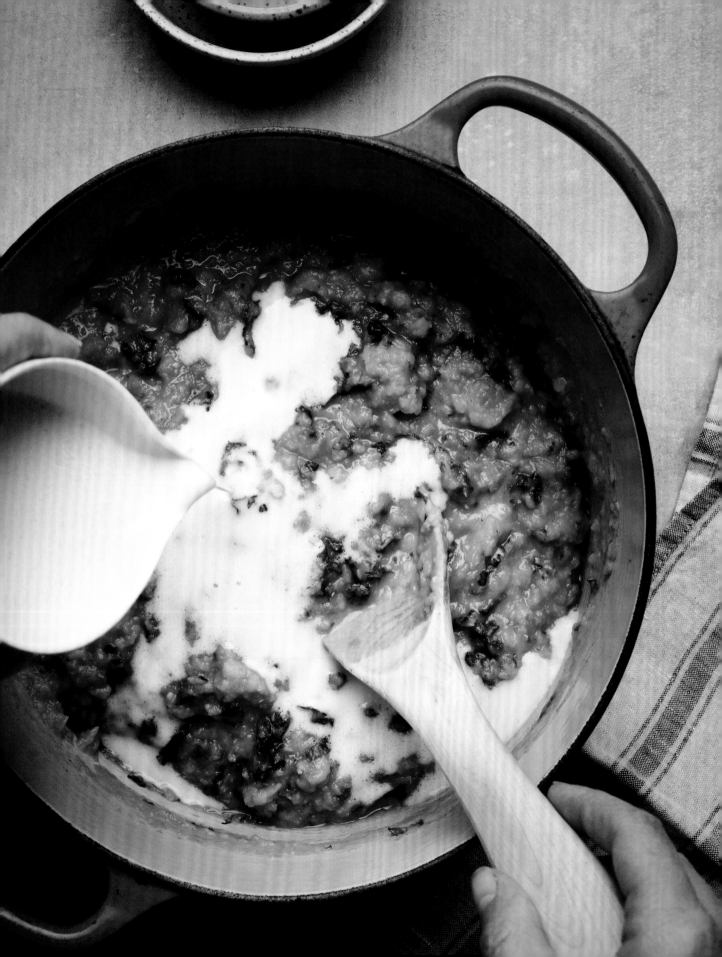

Red Lentil and Root Veggie Comfort Soup

⊕ **CALM, FOCUS, SLEEP, UPLIFT**

PREP TIME: 7 MINUTES **COOK TIME:** 35 MINUTES **SERVES:** 4

1½ Tbsp coconut oil

3 garlic cloves, sliced

1 tsp onion powder

1 tsp ground turmeric

1 tsp ground cumin

½ tsp ground cinnamon

½ tsp sea salt

2 carrots, peeled and diced

1 turnip, peeled and diced

2 sweet potatoes, peeled and diced

4 cups vegetable broth or bone broth of choice

1 cup dried red lentils, rinsed

½ cup full-fat canned coconut milk

2 cups finely chopped kale

Squeeze of lemon or lime, for serving (optional)

Handful of fresh cilantro leaves, for garnish (optional)

Sarah: I make this soup often on Sundays, especially during colder months, and have leftovers for lunches over the next few days. The nourishing ingredients, like the turmeric, sweet potatoes, and lentils, and the warming, comforting nature of this soup always makes me feel a little better when I'm stressed, exhausted, or just feeling down. We love red lentils for their high fiber content and plant-based protein, and the root veggies and kale provide B vitamins and magnesium—our favorite mineral that can help with relaxation and sleep.

1 Heat a large pot over medium heat and add the oil. Once the oil has melted, add the garlic and cook for 30 seconds or until fragrant. Stir in the onion powder, turmeric, cumin, cinnamon, and salt, then cook for 30 seconds or until fragrant.

2 Add the carrots, turnip, and sweet potatoes, toss to coat in the spiced oil, and then sauté for 3 minutes. Pour in the broth and red lentils, stirring to combine. Bring the mixture to a boil, then reduce the heat to low, cover, and simmer for 25 minutes or until the lentils are soft. Add the coconut milk and kale, and cook for 5 minutes or until the kale wilts.

3 Serve with a squeeze of lemon or lime juice, plus a sprinkle of cilantro, if you like. Store leftovers in an airtight container in the fridge for up to 5 days or in the freezer for up to 2 months.

½ cup freshly squeezed orange juice (about 2 oranges)

2 garlic cloves, minced

1 Tbsp white miso paste

2 Tbsp extra virgin olive oil

2 tsp maple syrup

2 tsp tamari

1 tsp grated ginger

1 (8 oz) block tempeh, cut in triangles

Coconut Milk Cauliflower Rice (page 181)

½ cup kimchi or sauerkraut, for garnish (optional)

¼ cup microgreens, sprouts, or fresh herbs of choice, for garnish

Miso Orange Tempeh

⊕ CALM, ENERGIZE, FOCUS, UPLIFT

PREP TIME: 5 MINUTES   **COOK TIME:** 30 MINUTES   **SERVES:** 2–4

This recipe is a double win for fermented ingredients—tempeh and miso support the good bacteria in your gut, helping you feel less stressed and more balanced. If you aren't well versed in cooking tempeh, this is an amazing recipe to start with because it's easy. The sweet orange and salty miso make a rich, complex marinade with just the right amount of spice from the fresh ginger and garlic. We love serving this with Coconut Milk Cauliflower Rice (page 181), but it's also perfect to add to salads, like our Ribboned Carrot Slaw with Miso Sesame Vinaigrette (page 175).

1   Preheat the oven to 375°F and line a small baking dish with parchment paper.

2   Whisk together the orange juice, garlic, miso, oil, maple syrup, tamari, and ginger in a small bowl.

3   Place the tempeh in the prepared baking dish, ensuring the triangles don't overlap one another. Pour the marinade overtop so it evenly covers all the tempeh. You can use your fingers here to turn the pieces of tempeh over to get all sides well coated.

4   Bake for 20 minutes, then flip each piece of tempeh over. You want the bottom side of the pieces to look a little crispy and lightly browned at this point. Bake for another 5–10 minutes, until the tempeh looks lightly browned at the edges.

5   Serve the tempeh overtop the cauliflower rice. Garnish with kimchi, if you like, and microgreens.

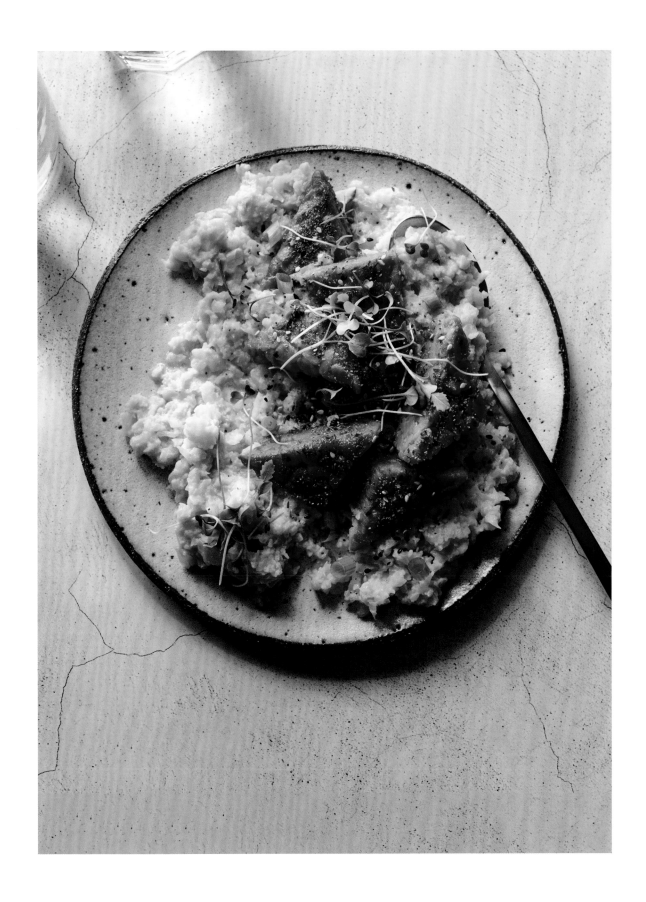

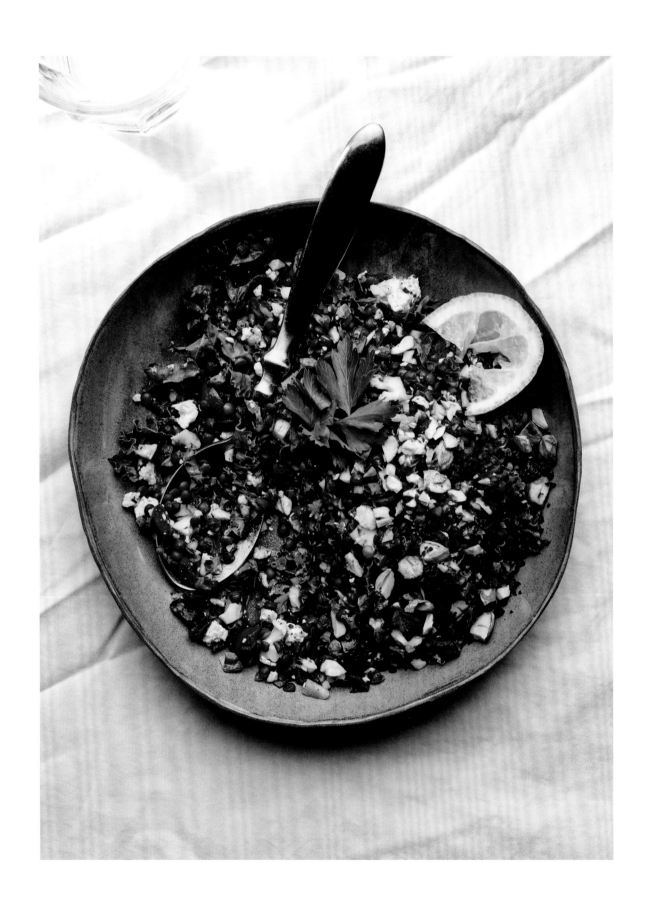

Lentil Crunch Salad

+ Blood Sugar Balancer

+ Colorful + Fiber-Rich

+ Healthy Fats + Prebiotic

+ Protein-Powered

1 cup dried beluga lentils, rinsed

4 cups water

½ tsp sea salt, plus a pinch

½ cup extra virgin olive oil

2 garlic cloves

1 lemon, zested and juiced

¼ cup roughly chopped fresh parsley

2 tsp sumac

⅛–¼ tsp red chili flakes (optional)

7 kale leaves, stemmed

½ cup finely chopped cauliflower florets

⅓–½ cup pitted kalamata olives, roughly chopped

⅓ cup crumbled feta, plus more for garnish (optional)

¾ cup pistachios, roughly chopped

⊕ CALM, ENERGIZE, FOCUS, UPLIFT

PREP TIME: 15 MINUTES   **COOK TIME:** 15–20 MINUTES   **SERVES:** 4

This salad has a lot going for it—zesty lemon, bright parsley, citrusy sumac, salty olives, crunchy cauliflower, nutty pistachios, and, of course, earthy lentils. We prefer beluga lentils for this recipe, since they're firmer than other varieties, but green lentils could work here too if that's what you've got. Lentils are one of the richest vegetarian sources of protein and also a fiber powerhouse, which will leave you feeling full, energized, and focused. You can pair this recipe with our Zucchini Pancakes with Miso Aioli (page 166), if you like.

1   Place the lentils, water, and pinch of salt in a medium pot. Leave uncovered, bring to a boil, and simmer for 15–20 minutes, until the lentils are tender yet chewy. Drain and rinse.

2   Place the oil, garlic, lemon zest and juice, parsley, sumac, ½ tsp salt, and chili flakes to taste in a blender or food processor and blend until emulsified. Alternatively, you can whisk the dressing in a bowl, but it emulsifies better when blended and the flavors heighten. If you're using the whisking method, first chop the parsley very finely and mince the garlic.

3   Roll the kale leaves up into a "cigar" and slice it into thin ribbons; transfer to a large bowl. Massage the kale with your hands for 30 seconds. Add the cooked lentils, cauliflower, olives, and feta to the bowl. Pour the dressing over and mix well. Top with more feta, if you like, and pistachios.

1 egg

¼ cup roughly chopped raw
walnuts

3 Tbsp roughly chopped
currants or raisins

1 lb ground beef

¼ cup finely chopped fresh
parsley

1 tsp garam masala

½ tsp ground cinnamon

½ tsp ground cumin

½ tsp sea salt

Pinch of pepper

¼ cup plain Greek yogurt or
dairy-free yogurt, for garnish
(optional)

2 Tbsp chopped fresh parsley,
for garnish (optional)

2 Tbsp pomegranate seeds, for
garnish (optional)

TAHINI LEMON SAUCE

3 Tbsp tahini

1½ Tbsp fresh squeezed lemon
juice

2 Tbsp cold water

Pinch of sea salt

Garam Masala Beef Keftas

⊕ CALM, ENERGIZE, FOCUS, UPLIFT

PREP TIME: 15 MINUTES   **COOK TIME:** 30 MINUTES   **SERVES:** 4

We are obsessed with these keftas, and so are our clients. They
have a wonderfully complex flavor while being very, very easy to
prepare. The garam masala makes this dish, so do not skip this
ingredient. The crunchy walnuts and sweet-yet-tart currants pair
really well with the beef. These keftas are high in protein, especially
the amino acid tryptophan, which can help you feel relaxed and
calm. Enjoy these with a salad, such as our Cucumber Salad Three
Ways (page 161), or with roasted veggies, such as our Blistered
Broccoli with Beet Tahini Drizzle (page 169).

1   Preheat the oven to 375°F or a grill to 350°F–400°F. If using the
    oven, line a baking sheet with parchment paper. If grilling and
    using 4–6 wooden skewers, soak the skewers in water for at least
    15 minutes so they don't burn on the grill. (Alternatively, you can
    use metal skewers.)

2   In a large bowl, whisk the egg. Add the walnuts, currants, beef,
    parsley, garam masala, cinnamon, cumin, salt, and pepper. Mix
    together until combined. It's easiest if you use your hands to do this.

3   **Roasting Method:** Form 3 Tbsp of the mixture into a football-shaped
    kefta. Place on the prepared baking sheet. Repeat with the
    remaining mixture. Bake for 20 minutes, then flip and bake for
    10 minutes more, until an inserted meat thermometer reads 160°F
    and the keftas are browned .

    Grilling Method: Shape the meat around the skewers into any shape
    you want—long logs or football-like shapes. Place the skewers on
    the grill and every few minutes flip using tongs. Cook for about
    10–15 minutes, until browned or until a meat thermometer inserted
    into the center of a kefta reads 160°F.

4   Prepare the sauce by combining the tahini, lemon juice, cold water,
    and salt in a bowl. Whisk until smooth and runny.

5   To serve, drizzle with the yogurt and sprinkle with the parsley and
    pomegranate seeds, if you like. Drizzle the tahini sauce overtop.
    Store leftovers in an airtight container in the fridge for up to 4 days.

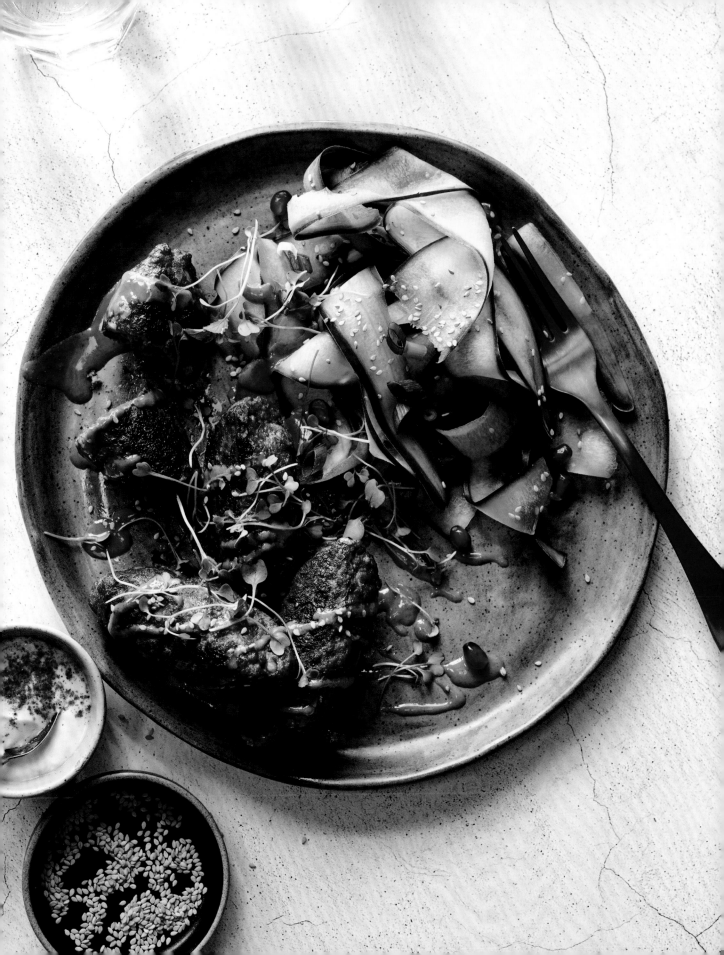

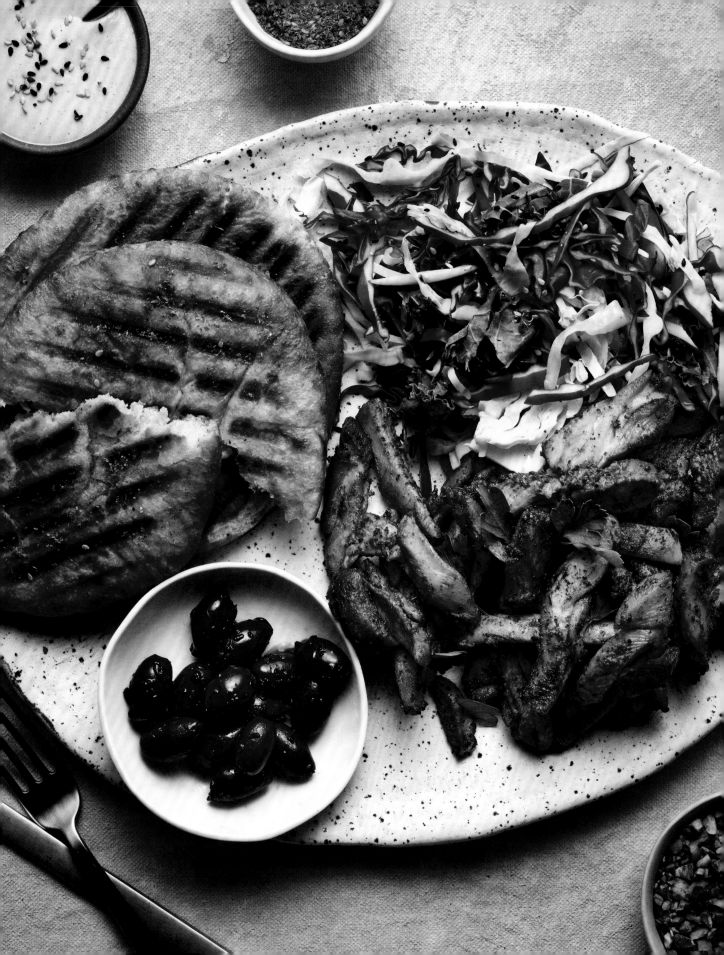

Crispy Turmeric Chicken Thighs

⊕ **CALM, ENERGIZE, FOCUS, UPLIFT**

PREP TIME: 15 MINUTES   **COOK TIME:** 30 MINUTES   **SERVES:** 4

1 lb boneless skinless chicken
   thighs

2½ Tbsp freshly squeezed
   lemon juice

¼ cup extra virgin olive oil

1 Tbsp sumac

1½ tsp ground cumin

1 tsp granulated garlic powder

1 tsp paprika

½ tsp ground turmeric

½ tsp sea salt

¼ tsp ground cinnamon

Pinch of pepper

¼ packed cup fresh cilantro,
   roughly chopped (optional)

Squeeze of lemon (optional)

This is one of our classic recipes—it's been in our repertoire for almost a decade. What makes this chicken particularly special—besides all the anti-inflammatory spices, like turmeric—is the broil at the end, which gives the chicken the perfect amount of crispiness. Chicken is a great source of the aminos acids needed to build your neurotransmitters, which stabilizes blood sugar and keeps you feeling focused and motivated as well as relaxed and calm. This recipe pairs well with many of our side dishes, like Crispy Brussels Sprouts with Homemade Labneh (page 162) or Rainbow Mediterranean Salad (page 165). You can also serve it with pita and olives.

1   Place the chicken, lemon juice, oil, sumac, cumin, garlic powder, paprika, turmeric, salt, cinnamon, and pepper in a large bowl, tossing to mix. Let the chicken sit in the fridge to marinate for 15 minutes or up to overnight.

2   Preheat the oven to 375°F and line a baking sheet with parchment paper.

3   Transfer the chicken to the prepared baking sheet and pour any marinade remaining in the bowl overtop. Bake for 25 minutes, until the internal temperature is 165°F; the exterior will be caramelized and slightly browned.

4   Remove the chicken from the oven, thinly slice and turn the oven to broil. Place the baking sheet on the center rack, so the parchment paper doesn't burn. Broil the chicken for about 2–4 minutes, until it gets really crispy but doesn't dry out.

5   Remove the chicken from the oven and arrange on a serving platter. Top with chopped cilantro and a squeeze of lemon, if you like.

Zucchini Mint Turkey Burgers with Cucumber Sumac Yogurt Sauce

⊕ **CALM, ENERGIZE, FOCUS, UPLIFT**

PREP TIME: 30 MINUTES + FREEZER TIME: 15 MINUTES
COOK TIME: 14 MINUTES **MAKES:** 4 BURGERS

These turkey burgers are great year-round, but especially during the warmer months. We often stuff veggies into our meat-based burgers to add extra flavor, texture, and nutrition (veggies add fiber here to support the good gut microbes, to help you feel happier). Enjoy with the Pretty in Purple Salad (page 176) or Apple Lime Walnut cucumber salad (page 161).

ZUCCHINI MINT TURKEY BURGERS

½ cup grated zucchini

2 Tbsp grated (or finely minced) red onion

1 lb ground turkey

1 egg

3 Tbsp finely chopped fresh parsley

3 Tbsp finely chopped fresh mint

½ tsp granulated garlic powder

½ tsp sea salt

Pinch of pepper

1 Tbsp extra virgin olive oil

CUCUMBER SUMAC YOGURT SAUCE

½ cup plain Greek yogurt or dairy-free yogurt

1 small garlic clove, minced

¼ cup grated cucumber

2 Tbsp freshly squeezed lemon juice

1 Tbsp finely chopped mint

1 tsp sumac

½ tsp sea salt

1 tsp honey

Pinch of pepper

TO SERVE (OPTIONAL)

4 burger buns

Butter lettuce or cabbage leaves

Roasted sweet potato disks (as buns)

Make the Burgers

1 Place the grated zucchini and onion in a cheesecloth, clean dish towel, or fine-mesh sieve and squeeze out the excess liquid.

2 In a large bowl, combine the turkey, zucchini, onion, egg, parsley, mint, garlic powder, salt, and pepper, mixing well.

3 Divide the mixture into four patties. Place on a plate, cover, and freeze for 15 minutes or refrigerate for up to 24 hours.

4 Preheat the oven to 350°F and line a baking sheet with parchment, or preheat a grill to 350°F–400°F.

5 **Stovetop/Oven Method:** Place a cast-iron skillet over medium heat, add 1 Tbsp olive oil. Once the oil is hot, place the patties in the pan, working in batches, don't overcrowd, and cook for 4–5 minutes per side. Place in the 350°F oven and bake for an additional 7 minutes, until the internal temperature reaches 165°F.

   Grilling Method: Cook the burgers for 5–7 minutes per side, until the internal temperature is 165°F, let rest for 5 minutes.

Make the Sauce

6 In a small bowl, combine the yogurt, garlic, cucumber, lemon juice, mint, sumac, salt, honey, and pepper.

7 Spread yogurt sauce on the bun or right on the burger if you're skipping the bun, and enjoy.

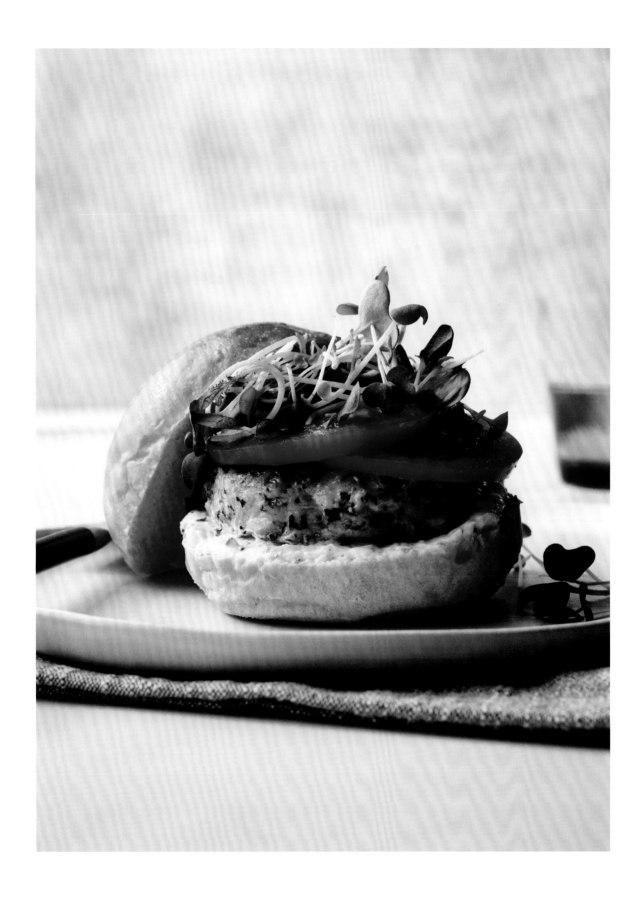

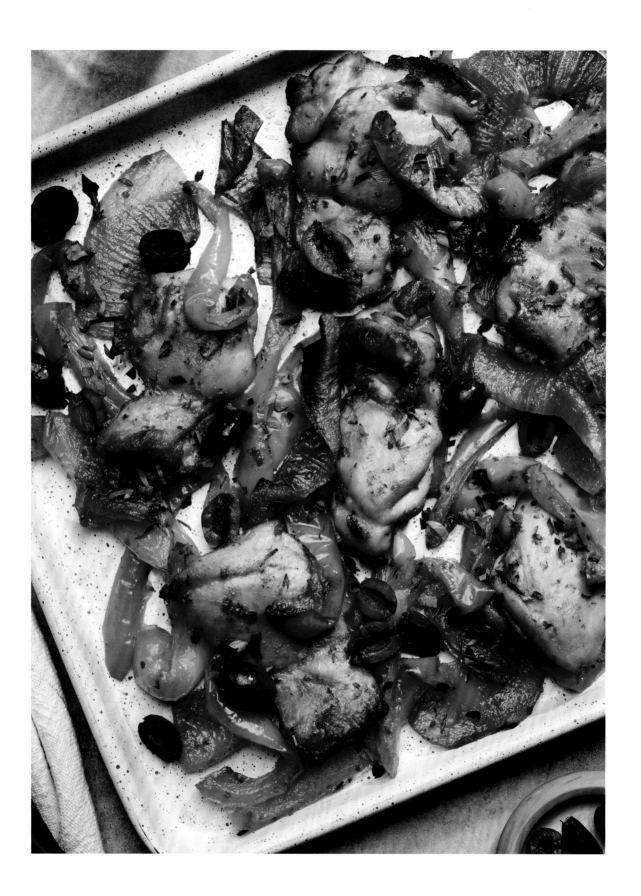

Sheet-Pan Lemon Chicken with Blistered Peppers

⊕ CALM, ENERGIZE, FOCUS, UPLIFT

PREP TIME: 20 MINUTES **COOK TIME:** 25–30 MINUTES **SERVES:** 2–4

¼ cup extra virgin olive oil

Juice of 1 lemon

2 tsp dried oregano

1 tsp paprika

1 tsp granulated garlic powder

½ tsp sea salt

A few cracks of pepper

1 lb boneless skinless chicken thighs

1 red onion, cut in thick half-moons

2 yellow bell peppers, thickly sliced

⅓ cup kalamata olives, pitted

¼ cup chopped fresh parsley, for garnish (optional)

Throughout this book, we ensure that the recipes are incredibly delicious, easy, and quick to make, knowing that most people are time-starved or simply do not want to spend hours in the kitchen. This Greek-inspired recipe may be one of our easiest! The chicken really only requires a quick marinade before being popped into the oven to do its thing. It's the perfect amount of salty (from the olives), lemony, and earthy (from the dried and fresh herbs), making this a tasty way to eat more protein to stabilize blood sugar and support feel-good neurotransmitters— ultimately helping you feel energized and focused. Enjoy this recipe on its own or with Super, Super Garlicky Greens (page 187) or Grilled Asparagus, Radish, and Potato Salad with Grainy Mustard Vinaigrette (page 170).

1   Preheat the oven to 375°F and line a baking sheet with parchment paper.

2   In a large bowl, whisk together the oil, lemon juice, oregano, paprika, garlic, salt, and pepper. Add the chicken, onion, and bell peppers, toss to combine, cover, and let sit in the fridge for 15 minutes.

3   Place the chicken mixture on the prepared baking sheet, spreading it out so as not to overcrowd. Roast for 25–30 minutes, flipping halfway through the cooking time. The chicken is cooked when its internal temperature reads 165°F; the chicken and peppers should be blistered and slightly browned. If they are not blistered, turn the oven to broil, and broil for 3–5 minutes. Watch carefully so nothing burns.

4   To serve, top the roasted chicken with the olives and parsley. If you would like to store the chicken for later, store in an airtight container in the fridge for up to 4 days.

Chicken Satay with Quickie Rainbow Slaw

⊕ CALM, ENERGIZE, FOCUS, UPLIFT
PREP TIME: 30 MINUTES **COOK TIME:** 25–30 MINUTES **SERVES:** 2–4

2 tsp coconut oil

2 Tbsp natural peanut butter or almond butter

1½ Tbsp Thai red curry paste

1 cup full-fat canned coconut milk (mix to combine solids and milk)

2 tsp coconut sugar

2 tsp tamari

1 Tbsp fresh squeezed lime juice

1 lb boneless skinless chicken breast, cut in 2-inch pieces

¼ tsp sea salt, plus more to taste

Pinch of pepper, plus more to taste

1 carrot, peeled and ribboned

½ English cucumber, ribboned

1 cup shredded purple cabbage

Juice of ½ lime

¼ cup toasted chopped peanuts or almonds

¼ cup mint leaves (optional)

NOTE: *If you don't have skewers or want to simplify things, skip the skewers.*

If you love Thai flavors, you must make this recipe. The satay sauce is undeniably delicious—you may be drinking it straight from the pot rather than pouring it over your meal! Adding a quick slaw rounds out the meal, and this perfect side dish takes just minutes to throw together.

1 Preheat the oven to 375°F and line a baking sheet with parchment paper, or heat a grill to 375°F–400°F. Soak six 8-inch wooden skewers in water (or use metal skewers) (see note).

2 Place a small saucepan over medium heat. Add the oil, once heated, stir in the nut butter, curry paste, coconut milk, sugar, tamari and lime juice. Mix until combined.

3 Thread 5 or 6 pieces of chicken onto the skewers, season with salt and pepper on all sides.

4 **Roasting Method:** Place chicken on the baking sheet, drizzle 3–4 Tbsp of sauce overtop, and roast for 20–25 minutes. The chicken will be slightly browned but not caramelized yet. Turn the oven to broil, move the baking sheet to a higher rack, and broil the chicken for 3–5 minutes, until parts of it are caramelized. The chicken is cooked when its internal temperature reads 165°F.

Grilling Method: With a bowl underneath to catch the drippings, pour 3–4 Tbsp of sauce over the chicken skewers. Place the skewers on the grill and cook for 10–14 minutes, flipping every 3–4 minutes, until the internal temperature is 165°F.

5 While the chicken is cooking, make the slaw by placing the vegetables in a bowl and toss with the lime juice, salt, and pepper.

6 To serve, place the slaw and chicken on a plate, and with a clean spoon, drizzle as much of the satay sauce as you like overtop both the chicken and the slaw. Garnish with nuts and mint.

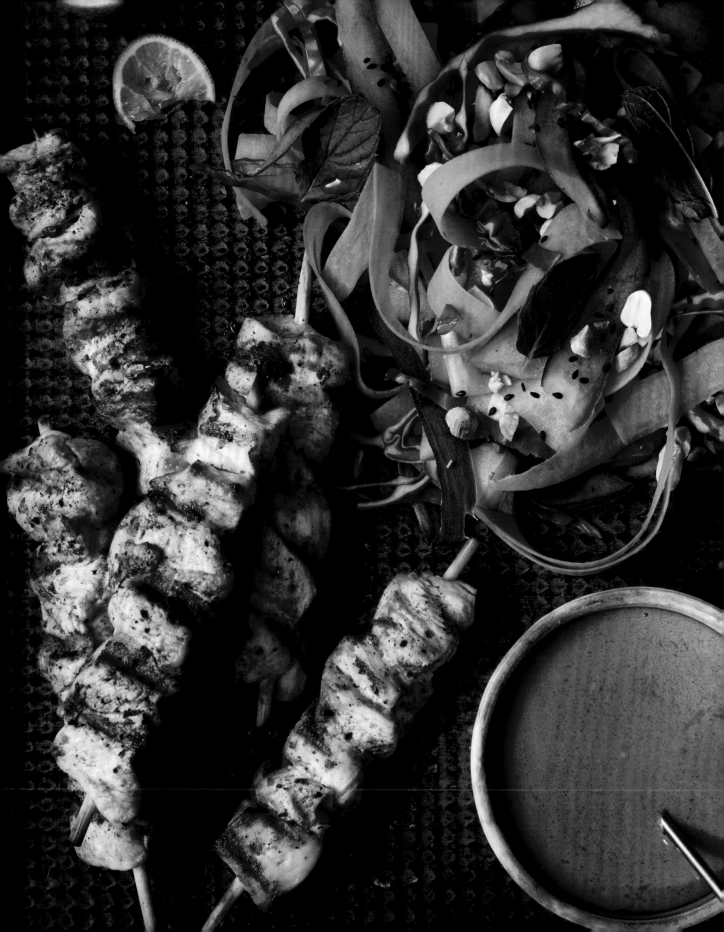

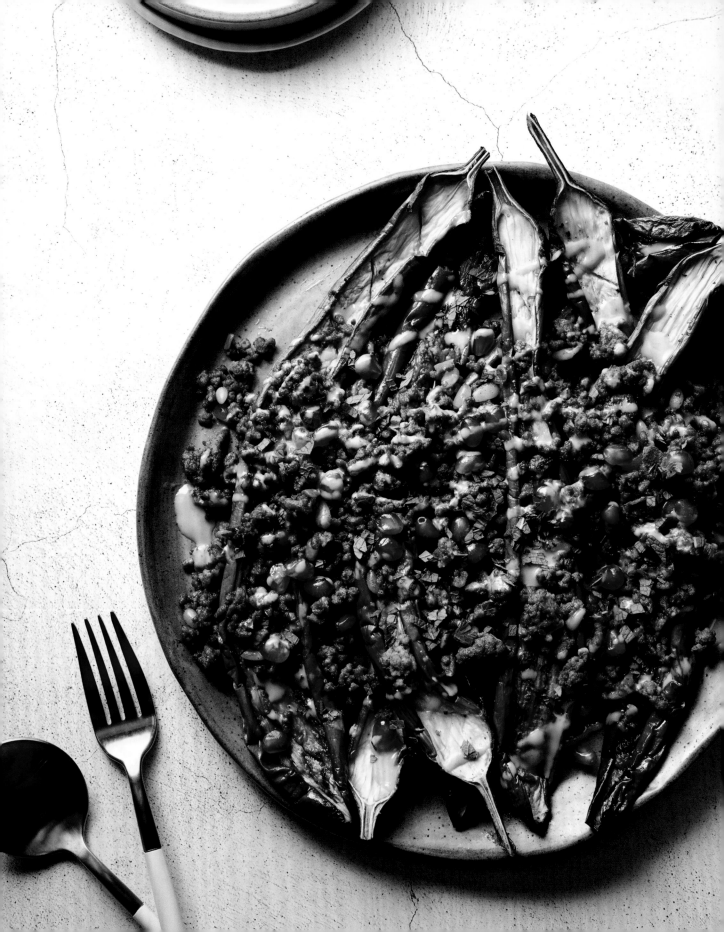

JAPANESE EGGPLANT

3 Japanese eggplant

1 Tbsp extra virgin olive oil

¼ tsp sea salt

A few cracks of pepper

SPICED BEEF

1 Tbsp extra virgin olive oil

1 small red onion, finely diced

1 tsp ground cumin

½ tsp ground coriander

½ tsp paprika

½ tsp sea salt

¼ tsp ground cinnamon

¼ tsp ground cardamom

Few cracks of pepper

1 lb ground beef

3 Tbsp pine nuts or slivered almonds

GARNISHES

Drizzle of tahini

Handful of fresh mint or parsley

2 Tbsp pomegranate seeds (optional)

NOTE: *If you can't find Japanese eggplant, you can use one large Italian eggplant (but since it's larger, you might need to roast it for longer).*

Spiced Beef with Japanese Eggplant

⊕ **CALM, ENERGIZE, FOCUS, UPLIFT**
PREP TIME: 10 MINUTES **COOK TIME:** 35 MINUTES **SERVES:** 4

This Middle Eastern–inspired dish is warming, deeply flavorful, and incredibly easy to make. Beef is rich in protein, which is needed to fuel the body and especially to feel energized and alert. It also helps build neurotransmitters in the body that elicit feelings of pleasure and happiness. We love the taste and texture of Japanese eggplant, but if you're not a fan, omit it and scatter the spiced beef over our Roasted Root Veggie Hummus (page 90).

Roast the Eggplant

1 Preheat the oven to 375°F and line a baking sheet with parchment paper.

2 Slice the Japanese eggplant in half vertically, then score the flesh by making diagonal cuts, but don't cut all the way through to the skin.

3 Place the eggplant on the baking sheet, flesh side up, brush it with oil, and season with salt and pepper. Roast for 30–35 minutes, flipping halfway through the cooking time. The eggplant is ready when the flesh is soft and golden brown.

Make the Beef

4 Place a large cast-iron or stainless steel skillet over medium heat, add the oil, then stir in the onion. Sauté for 5 minutes or until lightly browned.

5 Add the cumin, coriander, paprika, salt, cinnamon, cardamom, and pepper, stirring for 30 seconds to toast the spices before adding the beef. Break up the beef with a spoon, stirring to coat it in the spices, and cook for 7–10 minutes, until fully browned. Stir in the pine nuts. Remove from the heat.

6 To assemble, place the eggplant on a serving platter and top with the beef. Garnish with a drizzle of tahini, then toss the mint and pomegranate seeds overtop.

Chicken Salad with Pomegranate, Grapes, and Toasted Pecans

⊕ **CALM, ENERGIZE, FOCUS, UPLIFT**

PREP TIME: 10 MINUTES   **COOK TIME:** 15–20 MINUTES   **SERVES:** 4

2 boneless skinless chicken breasts

Pinch each of sea salt and pepper

2 Tbsp extra virgin olive oil

2 Tbsp freshly squeezed lemon juice

1 Tbsp whole grain mustard or Dijon mustard

2 tsp honey

½ tsp sea salt

A few cracks of pepper

1 cup thinly sliced kale

1 cup roughly chopped fresh parsley

½ cup halved purple grapes (about 10 grapes)

½ cup toasted pecans, roughly chopped

⅓ cup pomegranate seeds or dried cranberries

Drizzle of Beet Tahini Drizzle (page 169), for serving (optional)

We love making this salad for lunch—the natural sweetness of grapes is the perfect complement to nutty, toasted pecans and hearty kale. You'll find a rainbow of vegetables and chicken in this recipe, which means you'll get lots of fiber and prebiotics to fuel the good bacteria in your gut *and* protein to keep your blood sugar stable—this combo of nutrients will leave you feeling energized and focused, which makes this dish a great midday-meal option.

1   Place the chicken in a medium pot and cover with water. Add a pinch each of salt and pepper. Cover the pot, bring to a boil, and then simmer the chicken over medium heat for 15–20 minutes, until the internal temperature is 165°F.

2   Drain the water and rinse the chicken under cold water for a few seconds. Set aside until cool enough to shred with your hands or to slice into small pieces with a knife.

3   In a large bowl, whisk together the oil, lemon juice, mustard, honey, salt, and pepper. Add the chicken, kale, parsley, grapes, pecans, and pomegranate seeds. Toss well to combine.

4   Enjoy on its own or top with the Beet Tahini Drizzle. Store leftovers in an airtight container in the fridge for up to 4 days.

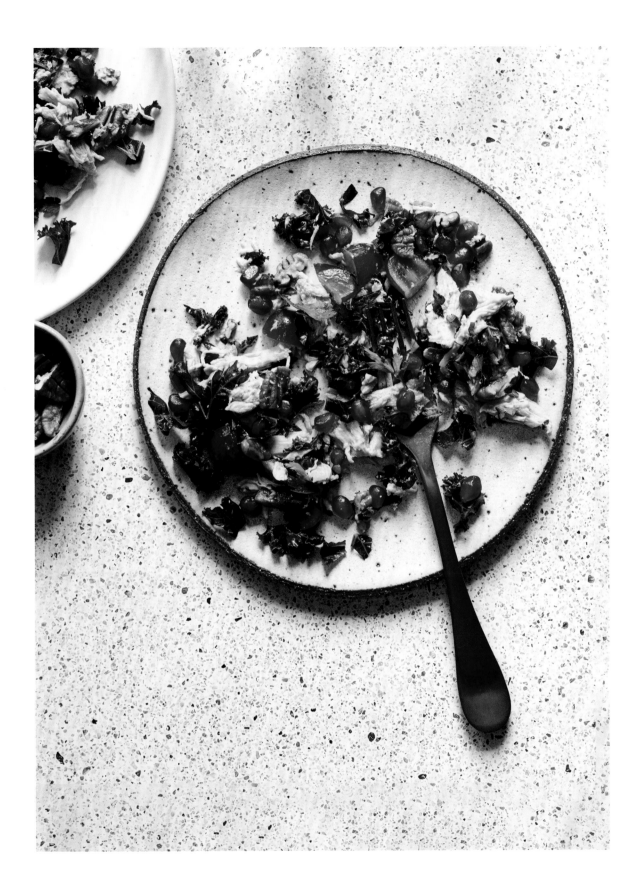

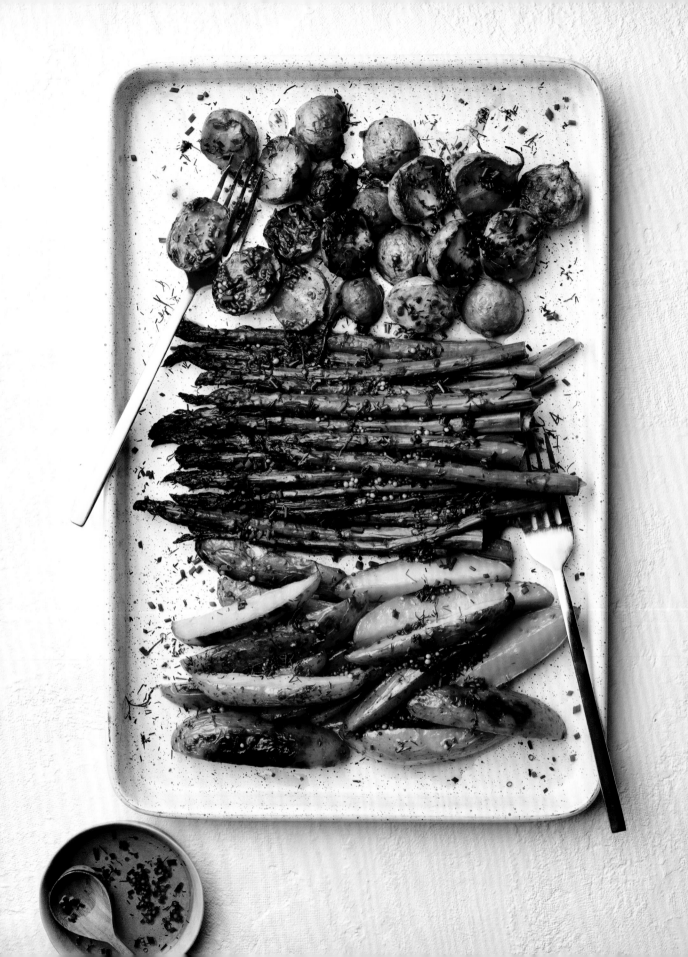

sides

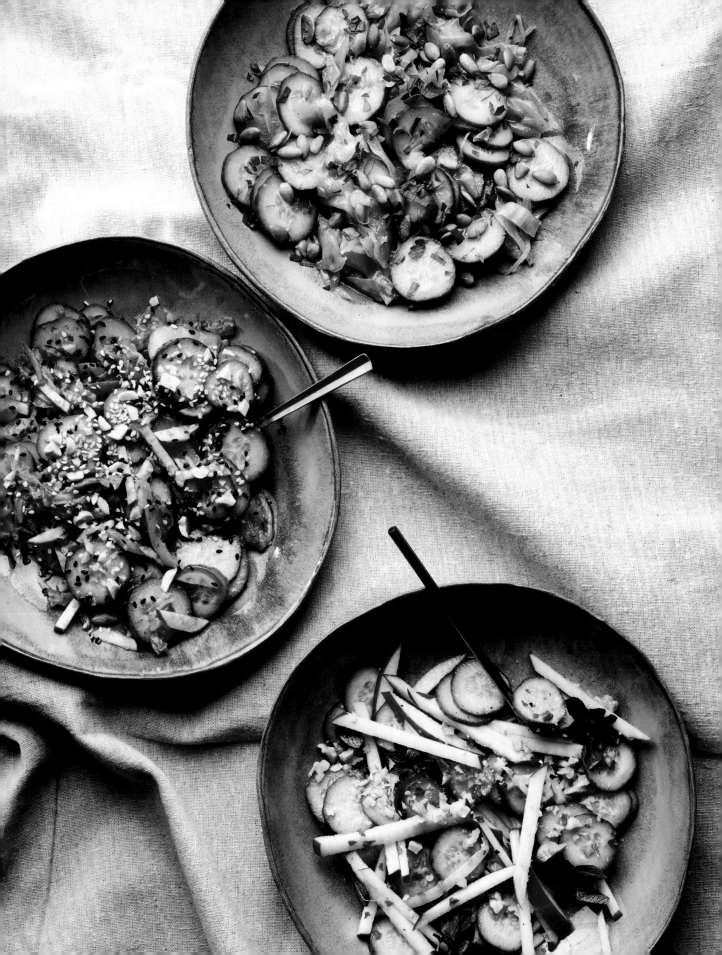

APPLE LIME WALNUT

4 Persian cucumbers, cut in
   thin rounds

1 crisp apple (such as Pink Lady,
   Honeycrisp, or Gala), cut in
   matchsticks

Juice of 1 lime (about
   2–2½ Tbsp)

1 Tbsp extra virgin olive oil

1 tsp maple syrup

¼ tsp red pepper flakes
   (optional)

¼ tsp sea salt

Pinch of pepper

¼ cup chopped toasted walnuts

**QUICK PICKLED WITH
FERMENTED CABBAGE**

4 Persian cucumbers, cut in
   thin rounds

1 Tbsp white wine vinegar

1 Tbsp freshly squeezed lemon
   juice

1 Tbsp extra virgin olive oil

½ tsp za'atar or sumac

½ cup sauerkraut

2 Tbsp toasted pumpkin seeds
   or pine nuts

SPICY SESAME AND PEANUT

4 Persian cucumbers, cut in
   thin rounds

4 small red radishes or
   1 watermelon radish,
   julienned

1 Tbsp rice vinegar

2 tsp extra virgin olive oil

2 tsp toasted sesame oil

½ cup kimchi

2 Tbsp toasted sesame seeds

2 Tbsp toasted peanuts,
   chopped finely

Cucumber Salad Three Ways

⊕ ENERGIZE, UPLIFT

PREP TIME: 10 MINUTES **SERVES:** 4

We love cucumber salads any time of year—in the summer they're refreshing and cooling, and in the winter they're a light and easy way to incorporate raw vegetables into our meals. Sauerkraut and kimchi both pair nicely with cucumbers, so this is a wonderful way to get more ferments onto your plate. These ferments support your gut microbes in a positive way, going on to help enhance cognitive function and improve overall mood. All cucumber salads are best eaten fresh, but if there are leftovers, they can be kept in the fridge to finish the next day.

Apple Lime Walnut

1 Place the cucumbers in a medium salad bowl and add the apple, lime juice, oil, maple syrup, red pepper flakes, salt, and pepper, and toss together.

2 Sprinkle the walnuts on top just before serving.

Quick Pickled with Fermented Cabbage

1 Place the cucumbers in a medium salad bowl and add the vinegar, lemon juice, oil, za'atar, and sauerkraut, and toss together.

2 Sprinkle the pumpkin seeds on top just before serving.

Spicy Sesame and Peanut

1 Place the cucumbers in a medium salad bowl and add the radishes, rice vinegar, oil, sesame oil, and kimchi, and toss together.

2 Sprinkle the sesame seeds and peanuts on top just before serving.

Crispy Brussels Sprouts with Homemade Labneh

⊕ **CALM, UPLIFT**

PREP TIME: 24 HOURS + 15 MINUTES   **COOK TIME:** 35 MINUTES
SERVES: 2–4

Labneh is a Middle Eastern cheese that is essentially strained yogurt. It's super thick, tangy, and creamy and has won our hearts. Brussels sprouts, a fibrous, vitamin B_6–rich veggie, turn deliciously tender and crisp once roasted. B_6 helps the body process stress more effectively. When serving this dish, ensure each spoonful has a bite of labneh, Brussels sprouts, and hazelnuts, for maximum flavor. This dish pairs well with our Crispy Turmeric Chicken Thighs (page 147).

LABNEH (SEE NOTE)

1½ cups plain full-fat yogurt or dairy-free yogurt

1 tsp freshly squeezed lemon juice

1 tsp sumac (optional)

¼ tsp sea salt

BRUSSELS SPROUTS

1 lb Brussels sprouts, trimmed and halved

1 small red onion, sliced thinly

2 Tbsp extra virgin olive oil

¼ tsp sea salt

A few cracks of pepper

TOPPINGS

¼ cup fresh mint leaves

¼ cup chopped toasted hazelnuts

1 Tbsp sesame seeds (optional)

Drizzle of honey

NOTE: *If you don't have time to make the labneh, you can replace it with a thick Greek yogurt.*

Make the Labneh

1 Place a fine-mesh sieve over a medium bowl, making sure the sieve is fairly high up and not touching the bottom of the bowl. Line the sieve with cheesecloth, a coffee filter, or a clean fine-weave dish towel. Scoop in the yogurt. Twist the top of the cheesecloth to close and then cover the bowl with a clean dish towel.

2 Refrigerate for 24 hours; the liquid will drain from the yogurt (full disclosure: your fridge will smell like labneh).

3 Scoop the labneh from the cheesecloth into a clean small bowl and stir in the lemon juice, sumac, and salt. Cover and refrigerate for up to 1 week until ready to use.

Make the Brussels Sprouts

4 Preheat the oven to 400°F. Line a baking sheet with parchment paper.

5 Place the Brussels sprouts and onion on the prepared baking sheet. Drizzle with the oil, and season with the salt and pepper. Toss to coat well.

6 Roast for 35 minutes, mixing the veggies halfway through the cooking time, until the sprouts are lightly browned and crispy at the edges.

7 To serve, spread the labneh on a serving platter. Top with the sprouts and onion, scatter the mint, hazelnuts, and sesame seeds overtop, and then drizzle with honey.

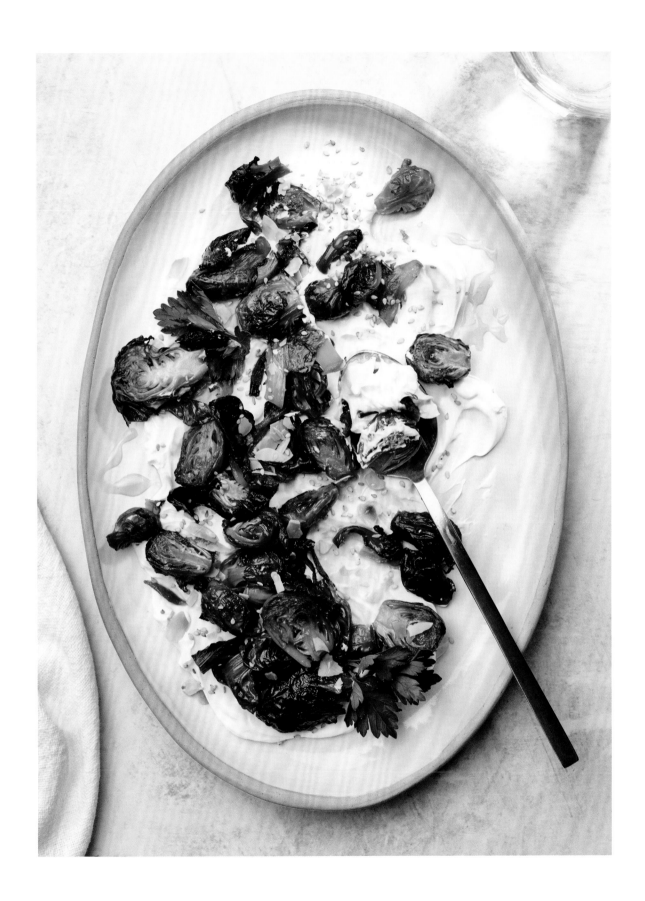

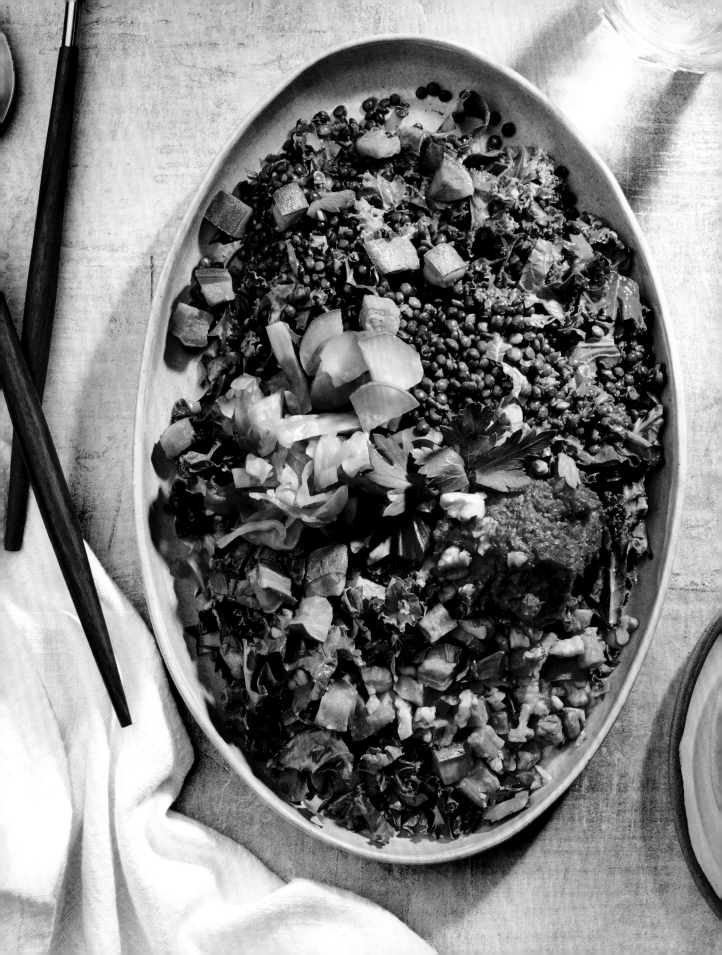

Rainbow Mediterranean Salad

1 large sweet potato, cut in ½-inch cubes

3 Tbsp + 3 tsp extra virgin olive oil, divided

Pinches each of sea salt and pepper

3 Tbsp freshly squeezed lemon juice

1 tsp maple syrup

1 small garlic clove, minced

1 cup cooked French or beluga lentils (see note)

1 small bunch green kale, stemmed and chopped

⅓ cup roasted walnuts, chopped

¼ cup chopped fresh parsley

¼ cup Beet Tahini Yogurt Dip, for garnish (page 88)

½ cup sauerkraut, for garnish

¼ cup chopped pickles, for garnish (optional)

✚ **CALM, UPLIFT**

PREP TIME: 15 MINUTES **COOK TIME:** 25 MINUTES **SERVES:** 4

This dish is inspired by a salad that we love eating from Parallel, a Toronto restaurant. It's fresh, a little sweet and salty, and has that crunch factor. This is the perfect recipe to ensure that you eat a rainbow of colors and lots of fiber to support the important bacteria in your gut, bacteria that have been shown to help increase mood and a positive outlook on life. We hope that when you eat this salad it'll make you feel like you're traveling to the Mediterranean, even though it's just in your imagination. This pairs well with Crispy Turmeric Chicken Thighs (page 147) and Hemp Mushroom Veggie Burgers with Thyme and Balsamic (page 128).

1 Preheat the oven to 375°F and line a baking sheet with parchment paper.

2 Spread the sweet potato on the prepared baking sheet, drizzle with 3 tsp of oil, and season with a pinch each of salt and pepper. Roast for 25 minutes or until tender and starting to crisp at the edges.

3 In a small bowl, whisk together the lemon juice, remaining 3 Tbsp oil, maple syrup, garlic, and a pinch each of salt and pepper to make the dressing.

4 Place the sweet potato, lentils, kale, walnuts, and parsley in a large bowl. Drizzle all the dressing overtop and toss to coat.

5 Just before serving, add a scoop of the yogurt dip, sauerkraut and pickles on top of the salad. This salad is best eaten right away, but if you have leftovers, you can store them in an airtight container in the fridge for the next day.

NOTE: *Place ½ cup of dried French or beluga lentils in a medium pot, cover with water, and add a pinch of salt. Leave uncovered, bring to a boil, and simmer for 15–20 minutes, until tender yet chewy. Drain and rinse.*

+ Blood Sugar Balancer
+ Colorful + Fermented
+ Prebiotic

4 cups grated zucchini (about 2 medium zucchini)

½ tsp sea salt

2 eggs, whisked

1 cup cooked quinoa (see note)

¼ cup oat flour

¼ cup chopped chives or green onions, plus more for garnish (optional)

¼ cup chopped fresh parsley, plus more for garnish

2 tsp extra virgin olive oil, plus more for cooking

½ tsp granulated garlic powder

½ cup mayonnaise (avocado oil or olive oil base)

2 Tbsp white miso paste

2 Tbsp freshly squeezed lemon juice

NOTE: *To cook quinoa, place ½ cup of quinoa and 1 cup of water, plus a pinch of sea salt, in a small pot. Bring to a boil and then cover, reduce heat to low, and simmer for 15 minutes or until quinoa is fluffy and the water is absorbed.*

Zucchini Pancakes with Miso Aioli

⊕ ENERGIZE, FOCUS

PREP TIME: 20 MINUTES **COOK TIME:** 30–35 MINUTES
MAKES: ABOUT 10 PANCAKES

These are a spin on a potato pancake, but a little greener! Eggs offer extra protein, which makes this a filling side dish that supports blood sugar stability, to help with focus, concentration, and steady energy. Although you may be tempted, do not skip the step of squeezing the liquid out of the zucchini, or the patties will be too wet. If you have leftovers, warming them up in the oven is a delicious way to dry them out and crisp the edges a little bit more. You can pair this with our Lentil Crunch Salad (page 143).

1   Preheat the oven to 400°F. Line a baking sheet with parchment paper.

2   Place the zucchini in a large bowl and sprinkle with the salt, mixing with your hands to gently combine. Let this sit for 10 minutes—the salt will pull the liquid out of the zucchini. After 10 minutes, transfer the zucchini to a fine-mesh sieve and squeeze or press the zucchini with your hands to remove the excess water. You'll be surprised by how much water comes out! The zucchini will reduce in size—you'll have around 2 cups now, instead of 4.

3   Place the zucchini, eggs, quinoa, oat flour, chives, parsley, oil, and garlic powder in a large bowl. Mix together to combine. You'll find the mixture is slightly liquidy—that's normal; it will stick together once cooked.

4   Drizzle a small amount of oil over the parchment paper to lightly coat it. Scoop out ¼ cup of batter and place on the baking sheet, gently pressing into a pancake shape. Repeat with the remaining batter. You should end up with about 10 pancakes.

5   Bake the pancakes for 25 minutes, then flip and bake for another 5–10 minutes, until the pancakes are lightly golden on top.

6   Whisk together the mayonnaise, miso, and lemon juice in a small bowl to make the aioli.

7   Serve the pancakes with the aioli and a sprinkle of chopped chives and parsley. Store leftovers in an airtight container in the fridge for up to 3 days or in the freezer for up to 2 months.

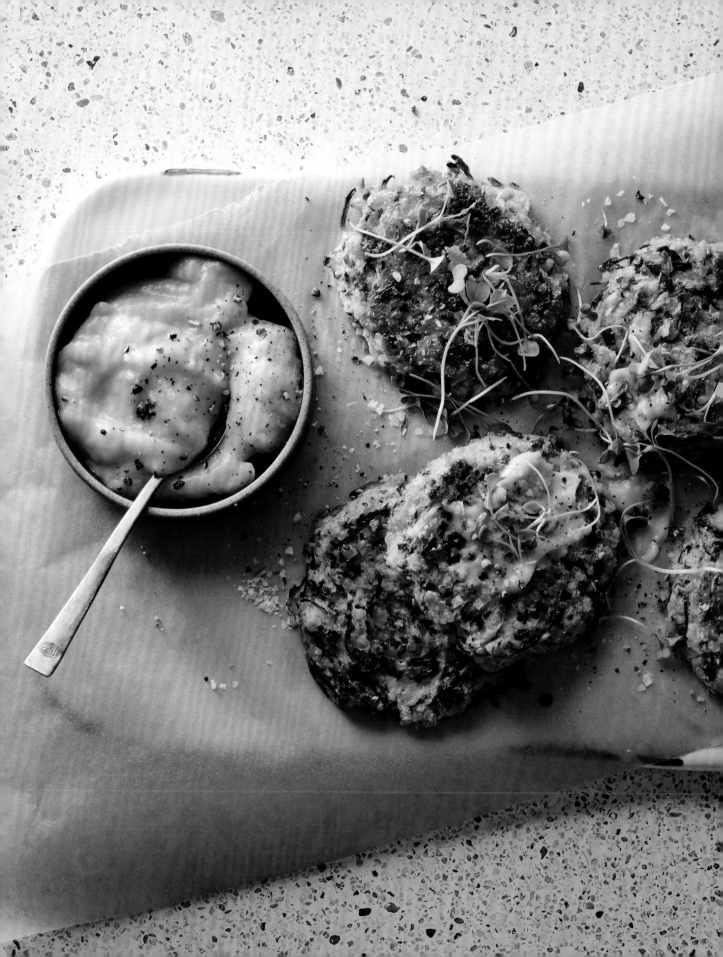

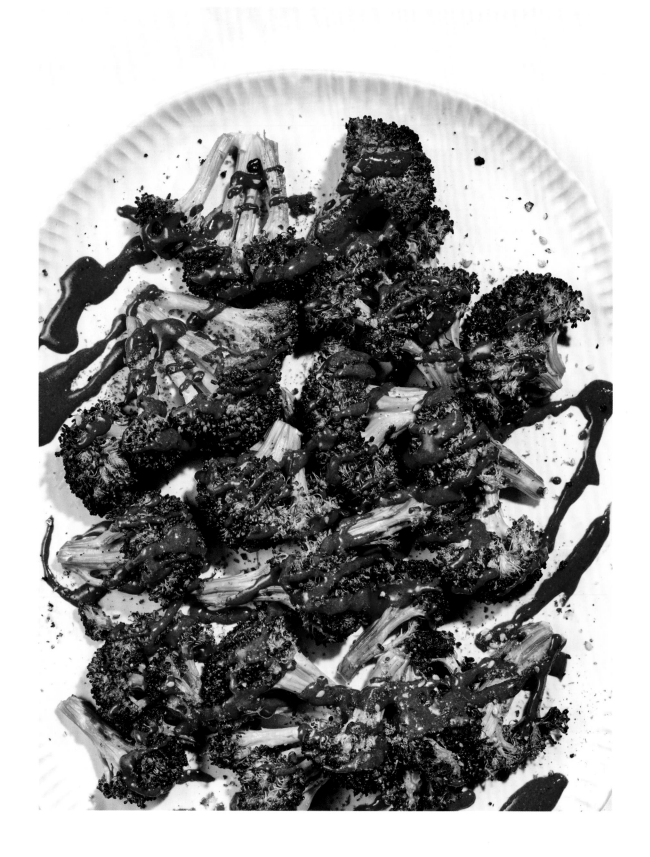

BROCCOLI

2 heads broccoli, cut in florets

2 Tbsp extra virgin olive oil

½ tsp granulated garlic powder

Pinch of sea salt and pepper

BEET TAHINI DRIZZLE

⅔ cup cooked cubed beets (see note)

⅓ cup tahini

2 Tbsp freshly squeezed lemon juice, plus more to taste

¼ cup cold water, plus more as needed

1 small garlic clove, minced

Pinch of sea salt, plus more to taste

GARNISHES

Sprinkle of za'atar

Sprinkle of sumac

NOTE: *You can use steamed, roasted, or even pre-cooked store-bought beets in this recipe. If you have any leftover cooked beets from another recipe, it'll work well here!*

Blistered Broccoli with Beet Tahini Drizzle

⊕ CALM, UPLIFT

PREP TIME: 10 MINUTES COOK TIME: 20 MINUTES SERVES: 4

Roasted broccoli trumps steamed broccoli by a long shot, elevating its texture and taste. The B-vitamins and powerful phytonutrients found in broccoli help relieve feelings of stress and anxiety. The beets in the tahini drizzle add color, sweetness, and fiber to fuel your microbiome, helping create more stable moods. You can serve this recipe with Garam Masala Beef Keftas (page 144).

1 Preheat the oven to 400°F. Line a baking sheet with parchment paper.

Make the Broccoli

2 Place the broccoli on the baking sheet, toss with oil, garlic powder, salt, and pepper to coat.

3 Roast for 20 minutes, until the broccoli is lightly crisp and browned at the edges and tender.

Make the Sauce

4 Combine the beets, tahini, lemon juice, water, garlic, and salt in a food processor and blend until smooth. Gradually add more water, a spoonful at a time, until the mixture's consistency is thin enough to drizzle over the broccoli. Taste and adjust the seasoning as needed—you may want to add more lemon juice or salt.

5 Remove the broccoli from the oven and place on a serving platter. Drizzle the beet tahini mixture overtop, or serve it in a side dish. Sprinkle za'atar and sumac overtop the broccoli.

Grilled Asparagus, Radish, and Potato Salad with Grainy Mustard Vinaigrette

⊕ **CALM, UPLIFT**

PREP TIME: 10 MINUTES **COOK TIME:** 35 MINUTES **SERVES:** 4

1 lb unpeeled fingerling
   potatoes or mini potatoes

1 bunch asparagus, ends
   trimmed

1 bunch radishes, trimmed and
   halved

4 Tbsp extra virgin olive oil,
   divided

Sea salt and pepper

2 Tbsp freshly squeezed lemon
   juice

1 tsp whole grain mustard

¼ cup chopped chives or green
   onions

2 Tbsp chopped fresh dill
   (optional)

NOTE: *If your potatoes are large, slice in half after they're cooked.*

Quick recap: prebiotics and resistant starches (found in asparagus and cooked, cooled potatoes) feed the good gut microbes—these veggies are good not only for your gut bacteria but for your taste buds too! Healthy gut bugs go on to make neurotransmitters, the ones responsible for feelings of happiness, pleasure, and relaxation. Asparagus is a seasonal vegetable in Canada and is abundant and fresh in the spring and summer. If you're eating this salad in the cooler months, replacing the asparagus with zucchini works perfectly. We like to pair this with our Sheet-Pan Lemon Chicken with Blistered Peppers (page 151).

1 Bring a medium pot of salted water to a boil. Add the potatoes and boil for 12–15 minutes, until you're able to pierce the potatoes easily with a fork, but they aren't falling apart. Remove from the heat, pour into a strainer, and run cold water overtop the potatoes for 30 seconds to cool them down enough to handle safely with your hands.

2 In a large bowl, use your hands to rub the potatoes, asparagus, and radishes with 2 Tbsp of oil and salt and pepper to taste.

3 **Stovetop Method:** Heat a grill-pan over medium-high heat. Cook the veggies for 5–7 minutes, then flip and cook for an additional 5–10 minutes, until the vegetables are tender and have light grill marks.

   Grilling Method: Preheat the grill to 375°F–400°F. Place the veggies in a grill basket and grill for 5–7 minutes, then give the basket a shake to move the veggies around. Cook for another 5–10 minutes, until the vegetables are tender.

4 Whisk together the lemon juice, the remaining 2 Tbsp oil, mustard, and a pinch of salt in a small bowl to make the vinaigrette.

5 In a large bowl, toss together the grilled veggies, chives, dill, and vinaigrette. Serve right away. Any leftovers can be stored in the fridge for up to 2 days. Serve cold or at room temperature.

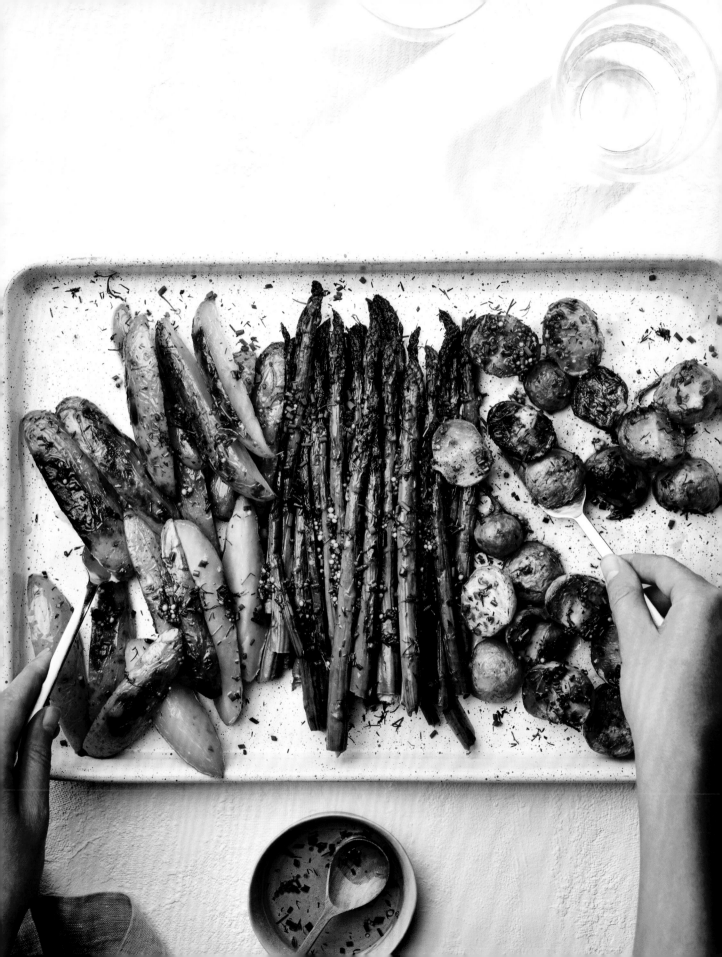

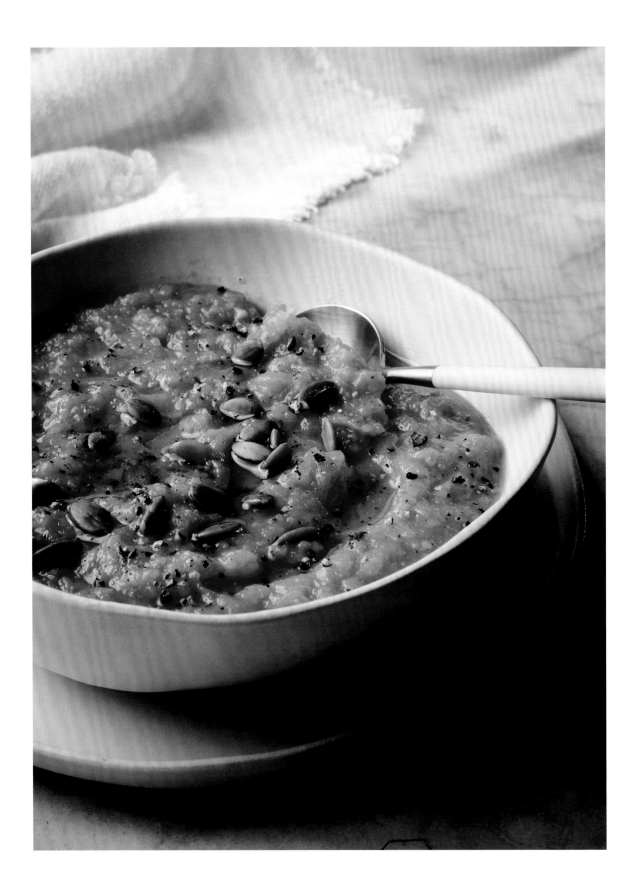

1 medium (2 lb) butternut
   squash, peeled, seeded, and
   cut in 1-inch pieces

3 medium carrots, peeled and
   cut in ½-inch pieces

3 Tbsp extra virgin olive oil,
   divided

¼ tsp sea salt

Pinch of pepper

1 shallot, diced

1-inch knob of ginger, peeled
   and roughly chopped

4 garlic cloves, thickly sliced

4 cups vegetable broth or bone
   broth of choice, plus more as
   needed

2 Tbsp white miso paste

4 Tbsp toasted pumpkin seeds,
   for garnish (optional)

Creamy Squash Miso Soup

✚ CALM, UPLIFT

PREP TIME: 10 MINUTES   COOK TIME: 45 MINUTES   SERVES: 4

When you think of miso soup, you may think of a soup that's traditionally served at Japanese restaurants. This soup offers the salty, umami flavor of miso, as well as its gut benefits, with the sweetness of roasted squash. All the veggies in this soup have their own unique flavor, including shallot, ginger, and garlic, which offer immune and prebiotic support. That helps good gut bugs flourish and in turn may help ease symptoms of depression and anxiety. This soup pairs well with our Crispy Chickpeas and Cauliflower over Lemony Tahini Yogurt (page 136).

1 Preheat the oven to 400°F and line a baking sheet with parchment paper.

2 Spread the squash and carrots on the baking sheet. Drizzle 1½ Tbsp of oil overtop, and season with the salt and pepper. You can use your hands to evenly coat the vegetables with the oil.

3 Roast for 25 minutes, then give everything a stir. Roast for another 20 minutes or until the squash begins to caramelize at the edges.

4 Ten minutes before the squash is ready to come out of the oven, place a large pot over medium heat and heat the remaining 1½ Tbsp oil.

5 Sauté the shallot in the hot oil for 4–5 minutes. When the shallot starts to become translucent, add the ginger and garlic. Sauté for 30 seconds or until fragrant.

6 Add the roasted squash and carrots to the pot, pour in the broth, stir everything together, cover, and heat to just below a boil.

7 Turn off the heat, add the miso, and using either a handheld immersion blender or a blender, blend until the soup is smooth and creamy. If the soup is thicker than you like, you can always add a little more broth or water to achieve your desired consistency. Season with salt and pepper, if needed.

8 Portion the soup into bowls and garnish each serving with 1 Tbsp pumpkin seeds. This soup makes for great leftovers. You can store it in an airtight container in the fridge for up to 5 days.

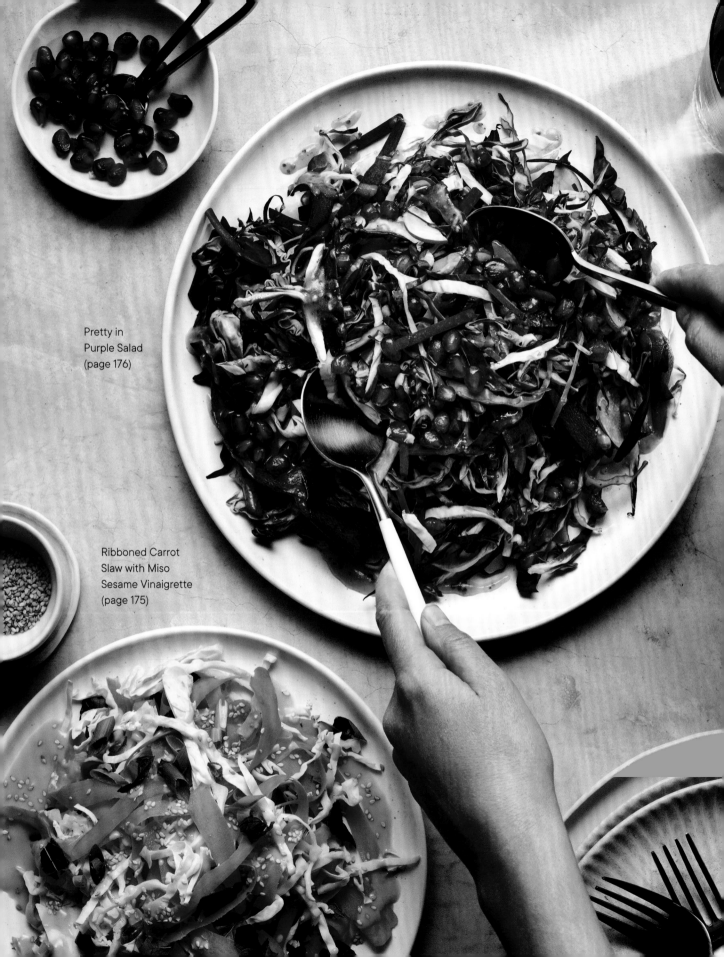

Pretty in
Purple Salad
(page 176)

Ribboned Carrot
Slaw with Miso
Sesame Vinaigrette
(page 175)

Ribboned Carrot Slaw with Miso Sesame Vinaigrette

⊕ **ENERGIZE, UPLIFT**
PREP TIME: 10 MINUTES **SERVES:** 4

1 lb carrots (about 6 medium carrots), peeled

2 cups shredded purple, green, or Napa cabbage

¼ cup mint leaves, torn

¼ cup fresh cilantro or basil leaves, torn

1 green onion, chopped

2 Tbsp toasted sesame seeds, plus more for garnish

MISO SESAME VINAIGRETTE

¼ cup extra virgin olive oil

2 Tbsp rice vinegar

3 Tbsp freshly squeezed orange juice

2 Tbsp freshly squeezed lime juice

1 Tbsp white miso paste

2 tsp chopped shallots

2 tsp toasted sesame oil

Pinch of sea salt

Ribboned carrots are beautiful and delicate—they'll make you feel like you ordered a gourmet dish from a restaurant, all while using a simple kitchen utensil (a vegetable peeler). We love dressing the carrots with this miso vinaigrette—it's savory but slightly sweet from the rice vinegar and orange, and a wonderful way to add that umami flavor to your salad. Eating more colorful plants, like the vegetables and herbs in this salad, has been shown to help boost moods. We like to pair this slaw with our Miso Orange Tempeh (page 140).

1 Using a vegetable peeler, pull from the top of a carrot down to the bottom, as if you were peeling it. Repeat this over and over, rotating the carrot as you go, until you've made as many ribbons as possible.

2 Place the carrot ribbons in a large bowl and add the cabbage, mint, cilantro, and green onion.

Make the Vinaigrette

3 Place the oil, vinegar, orange juice, lime juice, miso, shallots, sesame oil, and salt in a blender and blend until smooth.

4 Toss the vegetables with the dressing and sesame seeds. Serve with an extra sprinkle of sesame seeds, for garnish. Serve right away. Vinaigrette can be kept in the fridge for up to 5 days.

1 cup shredded purple cabbage

2 radishes, thinly sliced

1 small head radicchio, sliced

1 small purple beet, peeled and julienned

1 purple or orange carrot, peeled and ribboned

⅓ cup pomegranate seeds or dried cranberries

VINAIGRETTE

⅓ cup extra virgin olive oil

3 Tbsp red wine vinegar

2 tsp honey

1 tsp whole grain mustard

1 small garlic clove, minced

¼ tsp sea salt

A few cracks of pepper

Pretty in Purple Salad

⊕ CALM, ENERGIZE, UPLIFT

PREP TIME: 20 MINUTES SERVES: 4–6

Years ago, when we used to deliver meals to people's homes, this salad would often frequent the menu. It's strikingly stunning, with its vibrant purple and red palette, and offers your body all the protective polyphenol power that your microbes love, helping create neurotransmitters that influence your feelings of happiness and calm. If you are not a fan of radicchio, which is quite bitter, substitute it with more purple cabbage or dark kale. The vinaigrette includes red wine vinegar, which has been studied for its effects in lowering blood sugar, helping keep energy levels stable. This salad pairs well with our Sardine Pâté with Sourdough Toasties (page 121) or Zucchini Mint Turkey Burgers with Cucumber Sumac Yogurt Sauce (page 148).

1   Place the cabbage, radishes, radicchio, beet, and carrot in a large bowl.

2   For the vinaigrette, blend the oil, vinegar, honey, mustard, garlic, salt, and pepper in a small blender until emulsified. (If you don't have a small blender, simply whisk the ingredients together in a small bowl.)

3   Pour the vinaigrette over the vegetables, toss to mix, and top with pomegranate seeds. Store leftovers in an airtight container in the fridge for the next day.

Roasted Jerusalem Artichokes, Beets, and Cauliflower with Pistachio Dukkah

⊕ **CALM, UPLIFT**

PREP TIME: 20 MINUTES **COOK TIME:** 35 MINUTES **SERVES:** 4–6

Jerusalem artichokes are prebiotic superstars that are often overlooked. They are especially delightful when roasted with other vegetables and slathered in green tahini sauce and dukkah! The prebiotics in these veggies, especially in the artichokes, help feed the good bacteria in the gut—this improves immunity, reduces inflammation, and aids in stress relief. This is one of our more lengthy recipes but well worth making. It pairs incredibly well with our Orange-Infused Blackened Salmon (page 117).

JERUSALEM ARTICHOKES, BEETS, AND CAULIFLOWER

1 lb Jerusalem artichokes, unpeeled and scrubbed, cut in wedges

1 beet, peeled and cut in 8 wedges

4 cups cauliflower florets

3 Tbsp extra virgin olive oil

½ tsp sea salt

A few cracks of pepper

GREENISH TAHINI

1 small garlic clove, minced

½ cup creamy tahini

⅓ cup finely chopped fresh parsley

4–6 Tbsp cold water

2 Tbsp freshly squeezed lemon juice

¼ tsp sea salt

A few cracks of pepper

PISTACHIO DUKKAH

½ cup pistachios, finely chopped

2 Tbsp sesame seeds

½ tsp ground cumin

½ tsp coriander

½ tsp sea salt

Pinch of pepper

Roast the Vegetables

1 Preheat the oven to 400°F and line two baking sheets with parchment paper.

2 Spread the Jerusalem artichokes, beet, and cauliflower on the prepared baking sheets. Drizzle with the oil, season with the salt and pepper, and toss to coat. Roast for 30–35 minutes, stirring halfway through the cooking time. The vegetables are done when they're golden, softened, and slightly crisp.

Make the Greenish Tahini

3 There are two ways to make this dish—in a food processor or by hand.

Food Processor Method: Place the garlic, tahini, parsley, water, lemon juice, salt, and pepper in a food processor and process until the sauce is creamy and green.

By Hand Method: Stir together the garlic, tahini, parsley, water, lemon juice, salt, and pepper in a small bowl. This version will be more textured and less creamy than if made in a food processor but just as delicious.

CONTINUED

4 Place a medium skillet over medium-low heat, add the pistachios, and stir them occasionally until toasty, about 5–7 minutes (they'll continue to toast as the other ingredients go in). Turn the heat to low, add the sesame seeds, cumin, coriander, salt, and pepper and heat for another minute or until the spices are fragrant. If the pistachios begin browning too much, turn off the heat, but keep the pan on the burner and continue to toss for 30 seconds.

5 To serve, spread the tahini sauce on a serving platter, load the veggies on top, and sprinkle the dukkah overtop. Any remaining dukkah can be stored in an airtight container in the fridge for up to 1 month. Leftover veggies and the tahini sauce can be stored separately in airtight containers in the fridge for up to 4 days.

NOTE: *We adore the dukkah in this recipe, but if you're short on time, you can simply sprinkle toasted nuts or seeds (such as pistachios, walnuts, pumpkin seeds, or sunflower seeds) on top instead.*

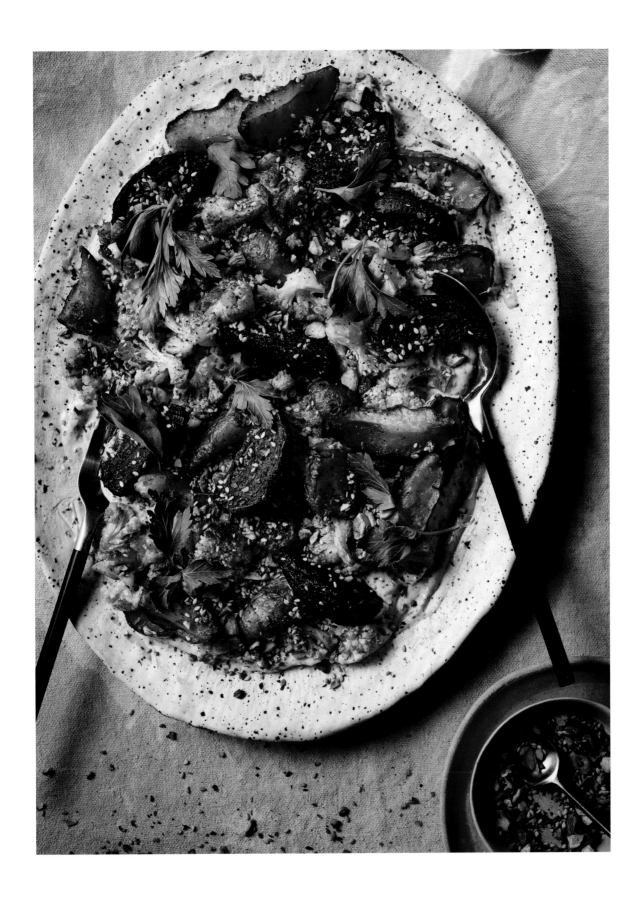

Golden Miso "Risotto"

⊕ **CALM**

PREP TIME: 10 MINUTES **COOK TIME:** 25 MINUTES **SERVES:** 2-4

1 cup quinoa

2 cups water

Sea salt and pepper

1 Tbsp butter or extra virgin olive oil

1½ cups sliced mixed mushrooms

1 leek, dark green part removed, rinsed well and thinly sliced

¼ cup white miso paste

3 Tbsp toasted sesame oil

1 Tbsp maple syrup

We should probably start by confessing that this isn't really risotto. But hear us out: the texture of this dish is risotto-esque—it's creamy, rich, warming, gooey. And another plus: you don't have to stand at a hot stove stirring for hours. This dish is one of our "classics"—possibly it's one of our oldest recipes that has stood the test of time. It's great to make on a dreary or cold day, or when you need some comfort, because the warming texture helps elicit feelings of calm and relaxation. You'll also get a good source of probiotics here from the miso, to support the friendly microbes in your gut.

1 Place the quinoa, water, and a sprinkle of salt in a medium pot, bring to a boil, cover, reduce heat to low and simmer for 15 minutes.

2 Meanwhile, place a large skillet over medium heat and add the butter. Once melted, add the mushrooms. Toss them in the butter, then cook for 5–7 minutes, until they release some liquid. Add the leek. Season with a pinch each of salt and pepper. Let the vegetables cook for another 15 minutes or until softened and slightly crisp.

3 In a small bowl, whisk together the miso, sesame oil, and maple syrup.

4 Add the cooked quinoa to the pan with the veggies. Turn off the heat, pour in the sauce, and stir well to combine.

5 Store leftovers in an airtight container in the fridge for up to 4 days.

Coconut Milk Cauliflower Rice

⊕ FOCUS, UPLIFT

PREP TIME: 5 MINUTES **COOK TIME:** 10 MINUTES **SERVES:** 4

1 head cauliflower, trimmed, or 1 bag (17.6 oz) riced cauliflower

1 Tbsp coconut oil

¾ cup full-fat canned coconut milk

Pinch each of sea salt and pepper

¼ cup chopped fresh herbs, such as cilantro or basil (optional)

This super simple recipe is probably the easiest way to enjoy cauliflower—it's just as quick as steaming it, but it's full of flavor and a little more exciting than its steamed counterpart. Although you may find that eating rice tends to send your blood sugar levels up, cauliflower "rice" is a great option for keeping meals lower on the glycemic index. It's a low-carb vegetable and is also a good source of fiber. The addition of coconut milk here makes this rich and creamy, rounding out the dish nicely. We love to serve this with our Miso Orange Tempeh (page 140) and One-Pan Miso Braised Cod and Leeks (page 122).

1 If you're using a head of cauliflower, cut it into florets. Place the florets in a food processor and pulse several times until the cauliflower is chopped up into tiny pieces resembling rice (you'll want to ensure that it has a coarse texture—don't overprocess it into mush).

2 Heat the oil in a large skillet set over medium heat. Add the riced cauliflower to the hot oil and sauté for 3 minutes to cook lightly—the cauliflower will still be firm at this point. Pour in the coconut milk, season with the salt and pepper, and stir to combine.

3 Cover and simmer over low heat for 7 minutes. Remove the lid and give the mixture a good stir. When it's ready, the cauliflower will be tender and some of the coconut milk will be absorbed. You can simmer with the lid off for a couple of more minutes, if needed. Add the herbs, if you like, just before serving. Store leftovers in an airtight container in the fridge for up to 4 days.

NOTE: *You can get creative with this recipe and use it as a base for stir fries—sauté some onions or garlic first, before adding in the cauliflower, if you like!*

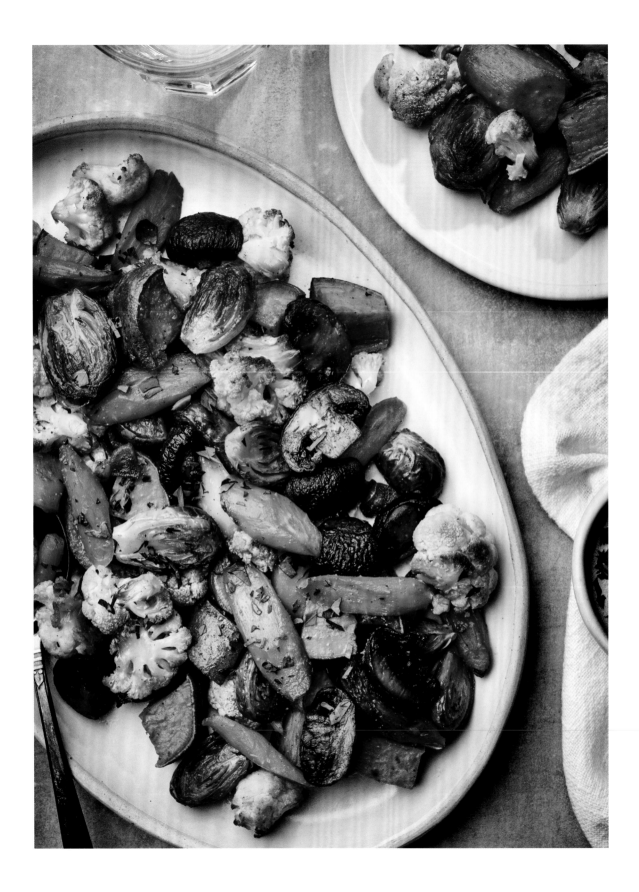

Our Favorite Roasted Veggie Medley

⊕ **CALM, UPLIFT**

PREP TIME: 20 MINUTES   **COOK TIME:** 35 MINUTES   **SERVES:** 6

1 lb sweet potatoes (about 2 medium), cubed

3 carrots, peeled and cut in ½-inch pieces

1 lb Brussels sprouts, trimmed and halved

1 head cauliflower, cut in florets

8 oz cremini mushrooms, halved

5 garlic cloves, sliced

4 Tbsp extra virgin olive oil

1 tsp granulated garlic powder

Pinch each of sea salt and pepper

1 red onion, sliced (optional, see note)

1 tsp dried Italian herbs or za'atar (optional, see note)

Roasted veggies are one of our go-to sides when making dinner, especially in the colder months when cooling salads are not as appealing. You can use any veggies you desire in this recipe, but our favorite combo is sweet, B-vitamin-rich root veggies to help with mood and stress, green veggies for phytonutrient powers, and mushrooms and garlic for prebiotics. Pair with our Hemp Mushroom Veggie Burgers with Thyme and Balsamic (page 128) or Green Herb Trout Burgers (page 118).

1   Preheat the oven to 400°F and line two large baking sheets with parchment paper.

2   Spread the sweet potatoes, carrots, Brussels sprouts, cauliflower, mushrooms, and garlic on the prepared baking sheets. Drizzle with the oil, and sprinkle with the garlic powder, salt, and pepper. Use your hands to rub the oil evenly onto the vegetables (you can always add a little more olive oil if the vegetables seem dry).

3   Roast for 25 minutes, then give everything a good stir. Roast for another 5–10 minutes, until everything is tender and edges of the carrots and cauliflower are starting to crisp. This is a great recipe to save for leftovers—store in an airtight container in the fridge for up to 5 days.

NOTE: *If you like onion or want extra flavor, add the optional ingredients. But these roasted veggies are so good all on their own too!*

Crispy Smashed Potatoes with Yogurt Sauce

⊕ **CALM, UPLIFT**

PREP TIME: 10 MINUTES **COOK TIME:** 45–50 MINUTES **SERVES:** 4–6

2 lb mini unpeeled potatoes (yellow, red, purple, any kind will do)

3 Tbsp extra virgin olive oil, divided, plus more to drizzle

1 tsp granulated garlic powder

1 tsp paprika

¼ tsp sea salt, plus more to season

Pinch of pepper

½ cup plain Greek yogurt or dairy-free yogurt

1 tsp lemon zest

2 tsp freshly squeezed lemon juice

A few Tbsp chopped fresh parsley

We could eat this recipe on repeat, weekly. It might sound simple, but those crispy edges of the potatoes, the subtle spice of garlic and paprika, and the cooling yogurt dip is the perfect combination. The protein and fat in the yogurt will help curb a major blood sugar spike, in turn helping prevent any feelings of sluggishness or low energy. Plus, pairing the potatoes with a protein-rich main, like our Orange-Infused Blackened Salmon (page 117), will help too!

1 Place the potatoes in a large pot, cover with water, and bring to a boil. Reduce the heat to low and cook for 15–20 minutes, until you can pierce the potatoes with a fork but they're still slightly firm.

2 Preheat the oven to 400°F. Drizzle a bit of oil over two baking sheets. Once the potatoes have been cooking for 15 minutes, place the oiled baking sheets in the oven to heat them up.

3 Mix together the garlic powder, paprika, salt, and pepper in a small bowl.

4 Drain the potatoes. Carefully take the baking sheets out of the oven and place the potatoes on them, making sure to not overcrowd them. You should hear a sizzle. Take the back of a glass and smash each one down—enough that it flattens, but not so much that it falls apart.

5 Sprinkle the spice mixture over the potatoes, then drizzle 2 Tbsp of oil overtop.

6 Roast for 15 minutes, then flip and roast for 15–20 minutes more, until the potatoes are completely crisp at the edges.

7 In a small bowl, whisk together the yogurt, 1 Tbsp of oil, lemon zest, and lemon juice to make the yogurt sauce.

8 To serve, top the potatoes with dollops of the yogurt sauce and sprinkle with parsley. Store leftovers in an airtight container in the fridge for up to 4 days (it's best to store the yogurt sauce in a separate container from the potatoes so that you can add it once the potatoes have been reheated).

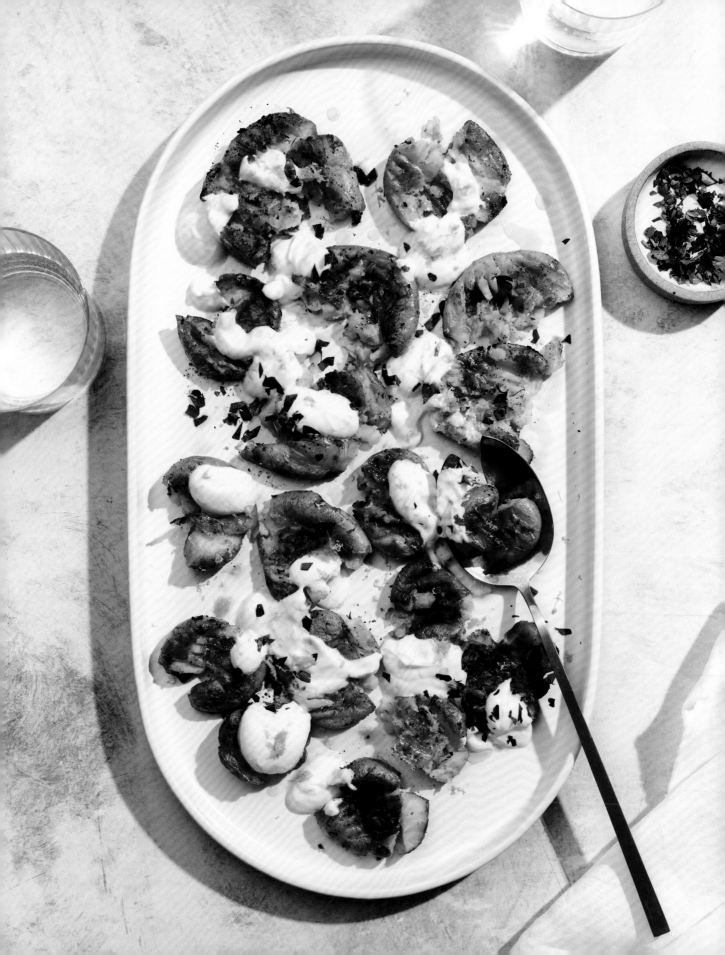

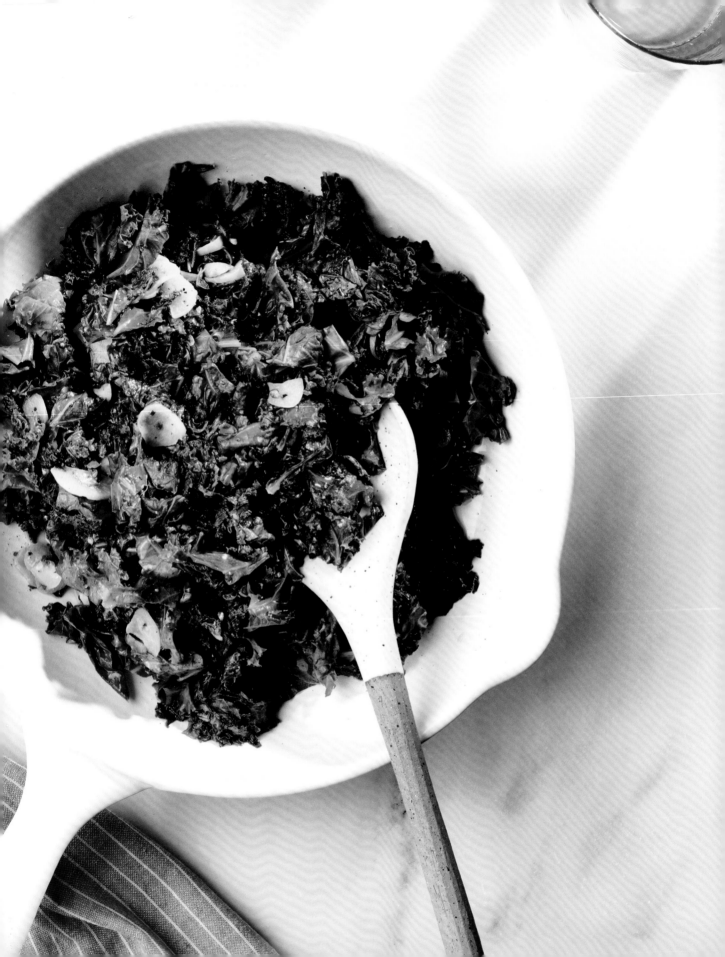

2 Tbsp extra virgin olive oil

6 garlic cloves, thinly sliced

1 big bunch (about 8 cups) kale, collards, chard, or bok choy (or a combo), chopped

¼ tsp sea salt, plus more to taste

A few cracks of pepper

1 Tbsp honey

Super, Super Garlicky Greens

⊕ CALM, UPLIFT

PREP TIME: 5 MINUTES **COOK TIME:** 10 MINUTES **SERVES:** 2–4

This is *the* recipe to make when you're short on time or need a quick side that requires minimal effort. You can use any greens you love, though we tend to stay away from spinach, since it wilts so much and results in a bit of a slimy texture. The high levels of magnesium in greens help boost feel-good chemicals and simultaneously calm the body. The combination of garlic, salt, and honey is all you need to make these greens tasty and special. It pairs exceptionally well with the Sheet-Pan Lemon Chicken with Blistered Peppers (page 151).

1 Place a large skillet over medium heat, add the oil, and swirl it around to coat the bottom. Add the garlic to the warm oil and stir until fragrant but not too browned, about 30 seconds (watch carefully so it doesn't burn).

2 Place the greens in the pan, add the salt and pepper, toss, then continue to cook the greens until wilted down for 5–7 minutes. Drizzle with honey and toss again. Season with sea salt, if needed.

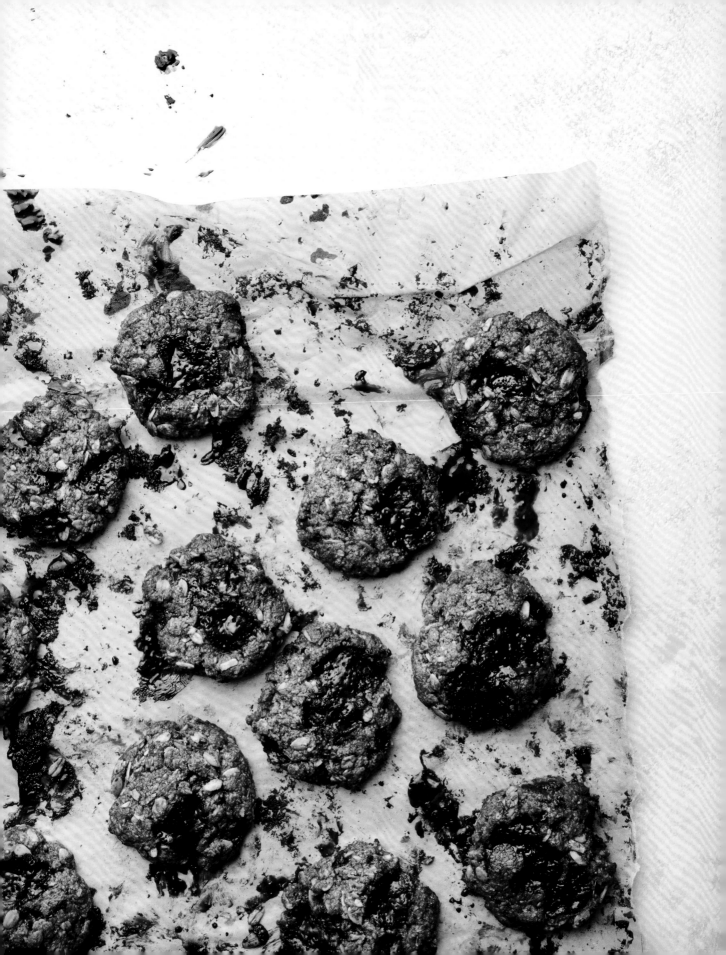

desserts

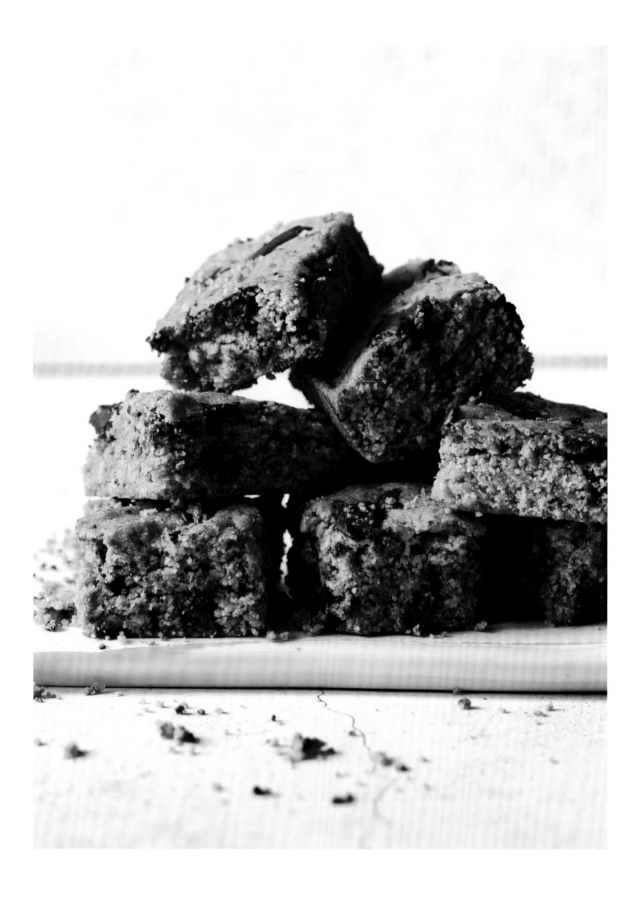

Almond Butter Blondies

⊕ UPLIFT

PREP TIME: 10 MINUTES   **BAKE TIME:** 23 MINUTES   **MAKES:** 10 BLONDIES

2 flax eggs (see note)

½ cup almond butter

2 Tbsp coconut oil, melted

½ cup coconut sugar

2 Tbsp maple syrup

½ tsp vanilla extract

½ cup oat flour

1 tsp baking powder

¼ tsp sea salt

¾ cup chopped dark chocolate bar or dark chocolate chips

We love almond butter in desserts—it's got that nutty, sweet, and creamy flavor we can't get enough of. So, naturally, we needed to combine it with dark chocolate to make a divine blondie that's perfectly chewy in the middle. Most desserts make you feel joyful when eating them, but they crash your blood sugar soon after, leaving you feeling tired and foggy. Almond butter is loaded with good fats and fiber—this helps stabilize blood sugar better, so you feel great during and after eating these blondies.

1   Preheat the oven to 350°F. Line an 8- × 8-inch baking pan with parchment paper.

2   Whisk the flax eggs in a medium bowl with the almond butter, coconut oil, coconut sugar, maple syrup and vanilla. In another medium bowl, mix together the oat flour, baking powder, and salt.

3   Fold the dry ingredients into the wet ingredients to combine; you'll find it's a very sticky batter. Stir the chocolate into the batter.

4   Evenly spread the batter in the prepared baking pan. Bake for 20–23 minutes or until firm on top and a knife or toothpick comes out clean when inserted into the center.

5   Remove from the oven and let cool in the baking pan for at least 15 minutes before slicing them. The longer they cool, the less crumbly they will be. You can store these in an airtight container in the fridge for up to 5 days.

NOTE: *To make the flax eggs, stir 2 Tbsp ground flax with 6 Tbsp of water in a small bowl. Let sit for 5 minutes until the mixture is slightly gooey.*

Probiotic Orange Creamsicles

⊕ ENERGIZE, UPLIFT

PREP TIME: 10 MINUTES **FREEZER TIME:** 6 HOURS **MAKES:** 9 POPSICLES

1¼ cups freshly squeezed
  orange juice

1 cup plain Greek yogurt or
  dairy-free yogurt

1 banana

1 Tbsp honey or maple syrup

1 tsp pure vanilla extract

These are citrusy, sweet, and packed with good-for-your-gut probiotic yogurt—which helps stabilize energy levels, making this a refreshing treat that fuels you up.

1 Blend orange juice, yogurt, banana, honey, and vanilla in a blender until smooth. Pour the mixture into popsicle molds.

2 Freeze for 30 minutes, then insert popsicle sticks. Freeze for 6 hours.

Coconut Berry-Swirl Popsicles

⊕ ENERGIZE, FOCUS, UPLIFT

PREP TIME: 15 MINUTES **FREEZER TIME:** 6 HOURS **MAKES:** 9 POPSICLES

1 can full-fat coconut milk

1 Tbsp honey

1 tsp pure vanilla extract

1 cup chopped strawberries

½ cup blackberries

A refreshing summer treat that combines polyphenol-rich berries with blood sugar stabilizing coconut milk. These popsicles look like a work of art and are the perfect, cooling treat.

1 In a blender, blitz the coconut milk, honey, and vanilla. Transfer most of the mixture to a container with a spout, leaving about ½ cup in the blender. Add the berries to the blender and blitz until smooth.

2 Divide the plain coconut mixture equally between the popsicles molds, filling up half-way. Pour the berry mixture overtop, and use a popsicle stick to gently swirl the milk and berries together.

3 Freeze for 30 minutes, then insert popsicle sticks. Freeze for 6 hours.

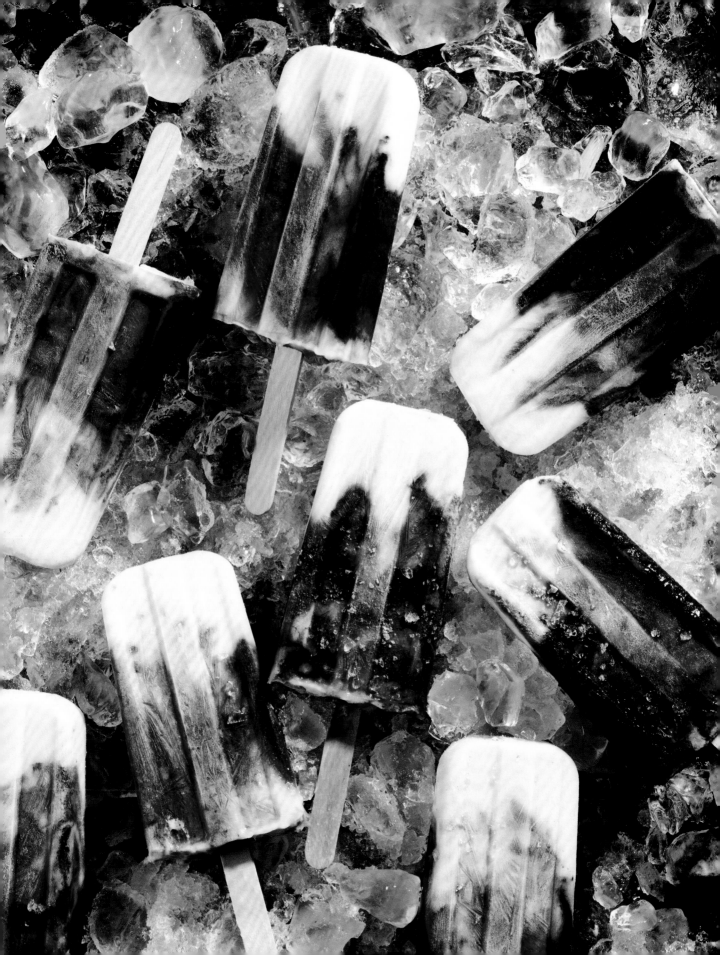

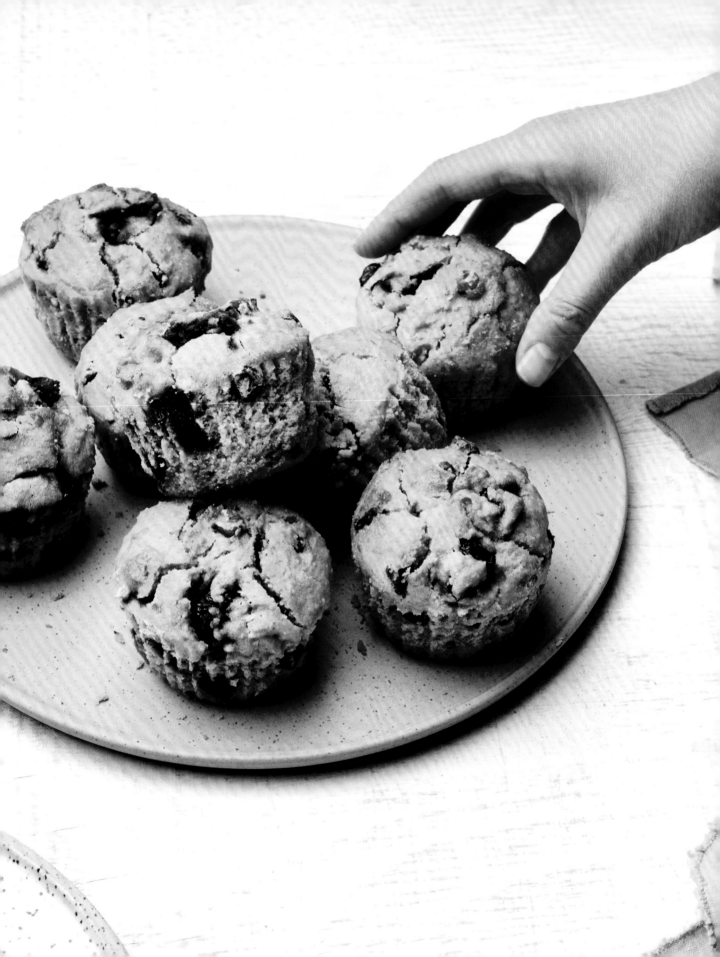

Dark Cherry Walnut Muffins

⊕ CALM, SLEEP, UPLIFT

PREP TIME: 10 MINUTES   **COOK TIME:** 30 MINUTES   **MAKES:** 12 MUFFINS

1 cup oat flour

1 cup almond flour

1 tsp baking powder

¼ tsp sea salt

2 eggs

½ cup milk of choice

¼ cup coconut oil, melted and cooled

¼ cup maple syrup

1 cup pitted and sliced dark cherries, fresh or frozen

⅓ cup chopped dark chocolate bar or dark chocolate chips

¼ cup chopped walnuts

We're always up for a muffin that's bursting with berries, crunchy nuts, and sweet chocolate. Did you know that drinking tart cherry juice has actually been shown to support better sleep?[64] Cherries are rich in melatonin, and while eating them won't deliver the same high concentration as the juice, you'll still get the polyphenol benefits—which supports a healthy gut and helps stabilize mood. Dark chocolate—our favorite—provides some magnesium to help support relaxation.

1   Preheat the oven to 350°F and line a muffin tin with 12 muffin liners.

2   In a large bowl, combine the oat flour, almond flour, baking powder, and salt. In another medium bowl, whisk together the eggs, milk, oil, and maple syrup.

3   Pour the wet ingredients into the dry ingredients, then fold together to combine. Gently stir in the cherries, chocolate, and walnuts.

4   Divide the batter evenly between the 12 muffin liners. Bake for 30 minutes or until a toothpick inserted in the center of a muffin comes out clean. Remove from the oven and let cool for 10 minutes before enjoying.

5   You can store the muffins at room temperature in an airtight container for 1 day and then in the fridge for up to 4 days. If you'd like to freeze the muffins, cool them completely and then pack in an airtight container and freeze for up to 2 months.

Almond Butter Chocolate Cups

⊕ **CALM, UPLIFT**

PREP TIME: 30 MINUTES **MAKES:** 5 LARGE CUPS

6 oz chopped dark chocolate bar or dark chocolate chips

2 tsp coconut oil

2 Tbsp natural creamy almond butter

Pinch of sea salt

Sprinkle of flakey sea salt (optional)

If you are a lover of easy desserts that combine almond butter and chocolate, this one's for you. These chocolate cups are very forgiving, so if you prefer to swap in peanut butter, tahini, or any nut or seed butter of your liking, they'll still be delicious. Your nervous system and blood sugar will thank you: thanks to the magnesium and glucose-balancing protein and fat, you'll avoid the post-dessert crash and feel perfectly satisfied instead. Don't you love it when something that tastes good is also good for you?!

1   Pour water into a small pot, 1–2 inches deep. Turn the heat to medium-low and place a heat-safe bowl overtop the pot, ensuring the bottom of the bowl is not touching the water. Add the chocolate and oil and stir every so often until they're melted. Carefully remove from the heat.

2   Line a muffin tin with 5 liners. Spoon 1 Tbsp of melted chocolate into each liner, then shake the tin to even out the chocolate. Place in the freezer for 10 minutes or until firm.

3   In a small bowl, stir together the almond butter and pinch of salt.

4   Spread 1 heaping tsp of almond butter over each portion of chocolate and return to the freezer for another 5 minutes.

5   Remove from the freezer and top each portion of almond butter with 1 Tbsp of melted chocolate. Shake the tin to even out the chocolate. Sprinkle with flakey sea salt and return to the freezer for 10 minutes or until firm.

6   Remove from the freezer and enjoy! You can store the almond butter chocolate cups in the freezer in an airtight container for up to 2 months (if they've been frozen for a while, let them sit at room temperature for a few minutes to soften a bit before eating).

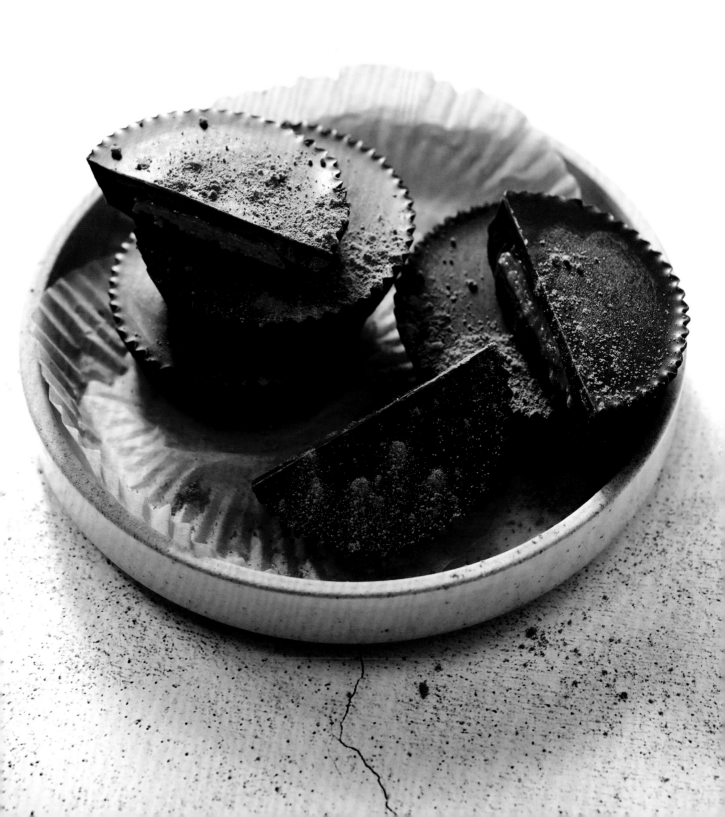

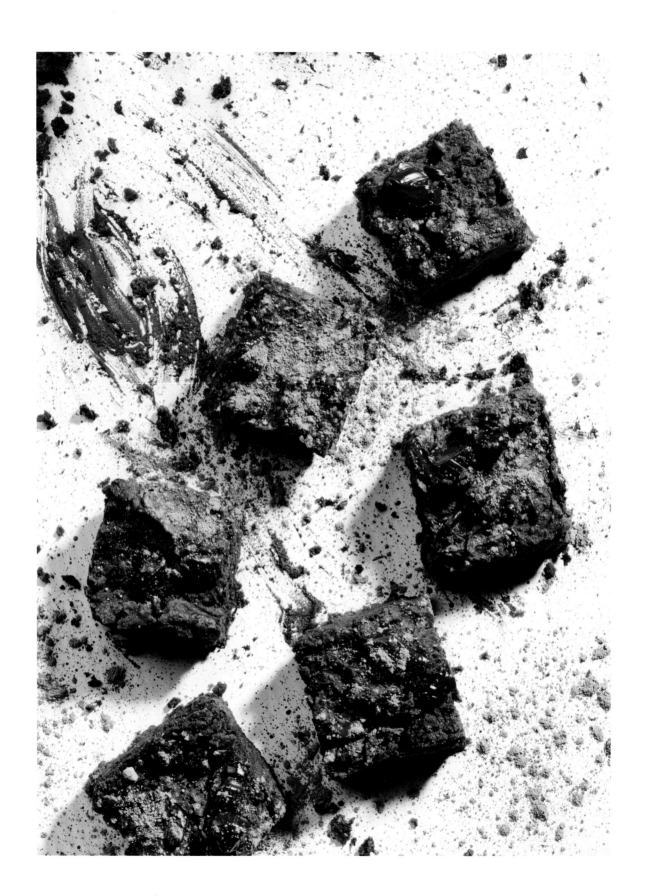

Fudgy Black Bean Brownies

⊕ **UPLIFT**

PREP TIME: 10 MINUTES **BAKE TIME:** 35–40 MINUTES
MAKES: 16 SMALL BROWNIES

1 can (19 oz) black beans, drained and rinsed

2 eggs

½ cup coconut sugar

⅓ cup melted and cooled butter or coconut oil

¼ cup cacao powder or cocoa powder

½ tsp baking powder

½ tsp pure vanilla extract

¼ tsp sea salt

½ cup chopped dark chocolate bar or dark chocolate chips

Black bean brownies became really popular in the early 2000s and we're bringing them back! These brownies are fudgy, super-duper chocolatey, *and*, because their base is black beans, they're loaded with fiber that feeds all those good gut bugs. A happy gut helps your body build neurotransmitters responsible for feeling joyful, optimistic, and satisfied. They will also be devoured very, very quickly. Who says desserts can't be fiber-rich?

1   Preheat the oven to 350°F. Oil an 8- × 8-inch baking pan and line it with parchment paper.

2   Place the black beans, eggs, coconut sugar, butter, cacao powder, baking powder, vanilla, and salt in a food processor. Process until smooth.

3   Pour the batter into the prepared baking pan, stir in the chocolate, then even out the batter using a spatula or spoon. Bake for 35–40 minutes, until a toothpick inserted into the center comes out clean.

4   Remove from the oven and allow to cool in the pan for 10 minutes, then slice them into 16 squares. Store in an airtight container in the fridge for up to 4 days.

CRUST

1 cup chickpea flour

½ cup almond flour or rolled oats

¼ tsp sea salt

3 Tbsp water

3 Tbsp melted and cooled butter or coconut oil

1 Tbsp honey

LEMONY TOPPING

1½ cups plain Greek yogurt or dairy-free yogurt

1 Tbsp + 1 tsp honey, divided

1½ tsp lemon zest

1 Tbsp freshly squeezed lemon juice

1 tsp pure vanilla extract

2 cups mixed berries of choice

A few spoonfuls of hemp seeds (optional)

Lemony Fresh Fruit Tart

⊕ **ENERGIZE, UPLIFT**

PREP TIME: 25 MINUTES **BAKE TIME:** 15–20 MINUTES **SERVES:** 4–6

A fresh, lemony fruit tart, especially in the heart of summer, is such a lovely dessert to enjoy. This crust boasts both fiber (from the chickpea flour) and healthy fats (from the almond flour). With the addition of probiotic and protein-rich Greek yogurt, plus colorful, polyphenol-powered berries, this is an incredible dessert for your blood sugar levels, gut bacteria, and taste buds. This means you'll feel perfectly satisfied and energized after eating it.

1 Preheat the oven to 350°F and line a 9-inch springform pan or a 9½-inch pie plate with parchment paper.

Make the Crust

2 Combine the chickpea flour, almond flour, and salt in a large bowl. Add the water, butter, and honey, mixing until a ball forms.

3 Place the dough in the prepared pan and, using your palm and fingertips, press the dough until it's evenly spread out. Poke it in a few places with a fork. Bake for 15–20 minutes, or until firm to the touch and slightly golden. Remove from the oven and allow to cool in the pan for 10 minutes, then remove the bottom of the pan.

Make the Topping

4 In a bowl, combine the yogurt, 1 Tbsp honey, lemon zest, lemon juice, and vanilla and mix well. Spoon the yogurt over the tart crust. Top with the berries and hemp seeds. Drizzle with the remaining 1 tsp honey. This dessert is best enjoyed immediately.

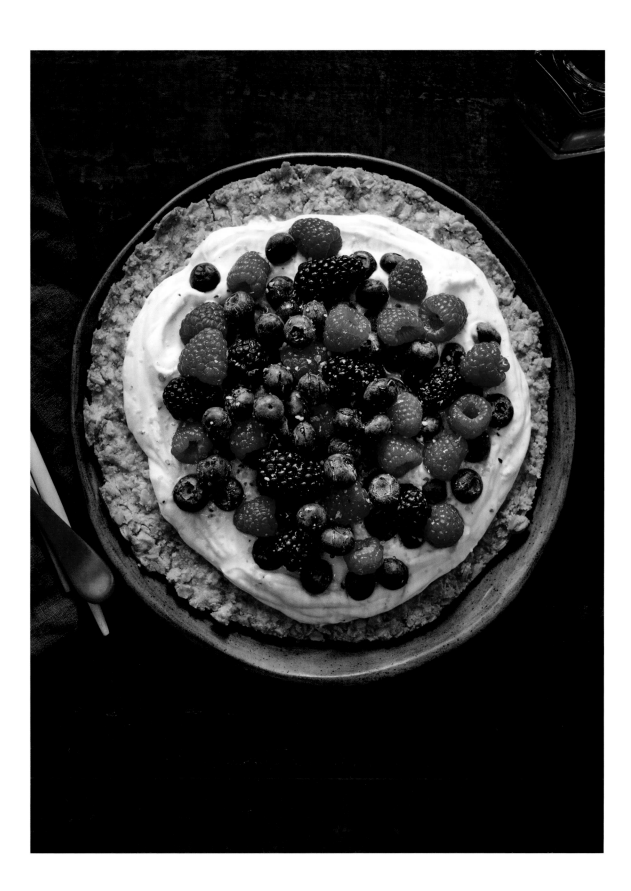

2 cups pitted and roughly sliced dark cherries (fresh or frozen)

4 Bartlett pears, cut in ½-inch cubes

1 Tbsp tapioca starch or arrowroot starch (see note)

2 tsp freshly squeezed lemon juice

1½ cups blanched, sliced almonds

1 cup unsweetened coconut flakes

¼ cup melted coconut oil or butter

2 Tbsp maple syrup

½ tsp ground cinnamon

Pinch of sea salt

Grain-Free Pear Cherry Crumble

⊕ **CALM, UPLIFT**

PREP TIME: 15 MINUTES   **COOK TIME:** 30 MINUTES   **SERVES:** 6–8

Crumbles and crisps have always been one of our go-to desserts, especially for dinner gatherings or picnics. This crumble is an easy dessert to whip up and never fails to deliver on flavor and appearance—you'll definitely want to scoop into the gooey, sweet filling when it's fresh out of the oven. If you don't have cherries readily available, feel free to swap in strawberries or any other combo of berries that you like. While cherries are thought to support sleep, you'll find lots of polyphenols in all types of berries, which help protect the brain.

1   Preheat the oven to 350°F and line a 1½ quart (6 cup) oval baking dish with parchment paper.

2   In a large bowl, toss together the cherries, pears, tapioca starch, and lemon juice to combine. In a separate large bowl, combine the almonds, coconut flakes, oil, maple syrup, cinnamon, and salt to make the topping.

3   Pour the fruit filling into the baking dish and spread out evenly. Spread the almond mixture overtop.

4   Bake for 30 minutes or until slightly golden on top and the fruit is bubbling. We love to eat this hot out of the oven, but you can store leftovers in an airtight container in the fridge for up to 4 days.

NOTE: *Both tapioca starch and arrowroot starch are grain-free and work as wonderful thickening agents instead of flour. If you don't have them, though, feel free to omit them here.*

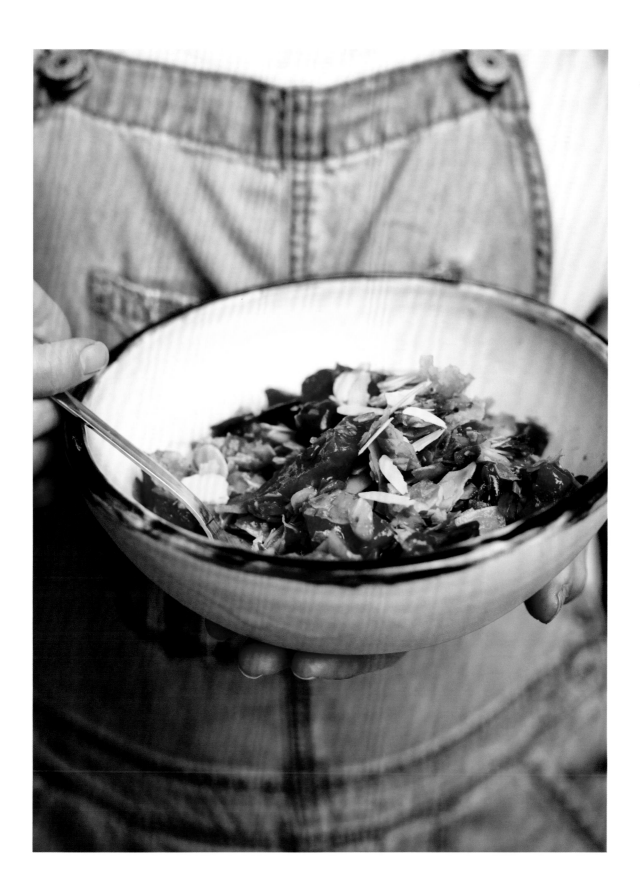

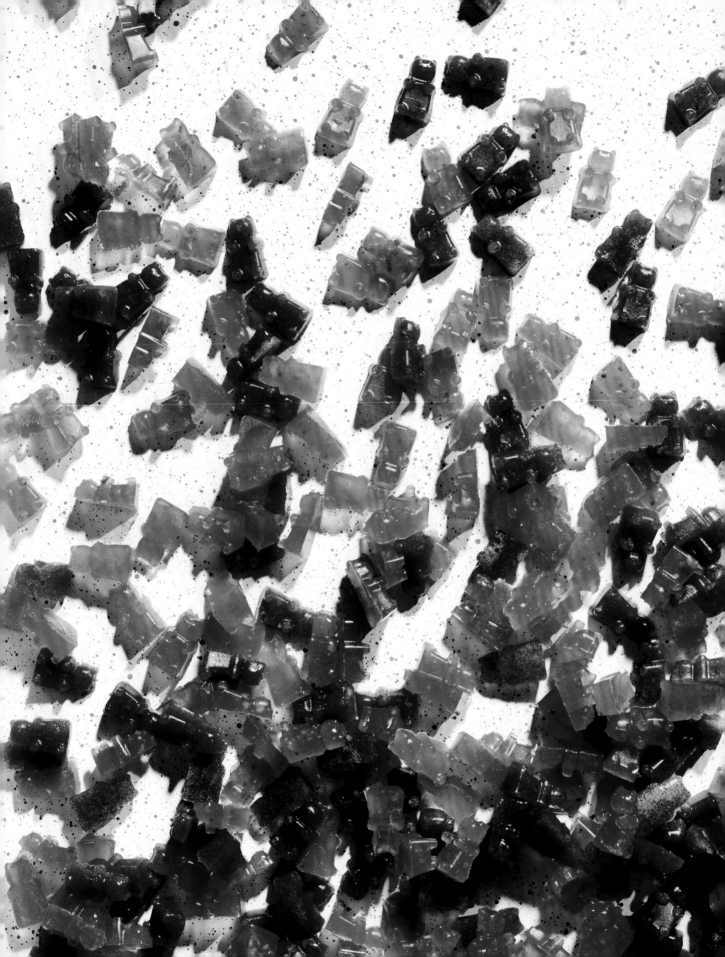

Berry Apple Gummies

⊕ ENERGIZE, FOCUS, UPLIFT

PREP TIME: 20 MINUTES **FRIDGE TIME:** 1–2 HOURS
MAKES: 740 SMALL GUMMIES

1¼ cups apple juice, divided

1 cup water

½ cup grass-fed gelatin (see note)

1½ cups chopped strawberries

½ cup blueberries or raspberries

2 Tbsp maple syrup

1 Tbsp freshly squeezed lemon juice

Did you love gummy bears as a kid? Get ready for a grown-up version that is fun to eat and good for you (these are totally kid-friendly too!). Gelatin, which gives things that gummy texture, is high in protein, so you can have a sweet treat that helps stabilize blood sugar. A quick reminder: you will need gummy molds to make these gummies; you can find them online or at kitchen stores.

1 Pour 1 cup of apple juice and the water into a large bowl. Whisk in the gelatin until combined. Let the mixture stand for 5 minutes.

2 In a blender, blend the strawberries, blueberries, maple syrup, lemon juice, and the remaining ¼ cup juice until the mixture is a smooth liquid.

3 Pour the berry mixture into a medium pot and set over low heat. Add the gelatin mixture and stir until it fully dissolves, about 2 minutes. Turn off the heat once it's liquid.

4 Use a gummy dropper, syringe, or small spoon to transfer the liquid into the gummy molds. Refrigerate for 1–2 hours, until the gummies have hardened. Remove from the molds and store in an airtight container in the fridge for up to 5 days.

NOTE: *You'll find grass-fed gelatin at any health food store or online. Also, if you prefer a sweeter gummy, you can add an additional 1–2 Tbsp of maple syrup.*

1½ cups roasted walnuts

1½ cups rolled oats

8 Medjool dates, pitted

¼ cup cacao powder or cocoa powder

3 Tbsp water

Pinch of sea salt

¾ cup dark chocolate chips or roughly chopped dark chocolate bar

2 tsp coconut oil

Sprinkle of flakey sea salt

Salty Chocolate Walnut Bars

⊕ CALM, UPLIFT

PREP TIME: 15 MINUTES **FRIDGE TIME:** 30 MINUTES **MAKES:** 10–12 BARS

These salty, crunchy, nutty bars will please every chocolate-loving taste bud you have—think of them as a healthier homemade chocolate bar. The base is dates and oats, which can spike blood sugar fairly high, but pairing them with walnuts helps keep your blood sugar a little more stable, so you won't feel the post-chocolate bar crash. The flakey salt on top is not to be missed.

1   Place the walnuts and oats in a food processor and process until a crumbly mixture forms. Add the dates, cacao powder, water, and salt and process until sticky.

2   Line a 10- × 5-inch loaf pan with parchment paper, and press the mixture into the pan to form the crust (or an 8- × 8-inch baking pan—use what you've got!)

3   To melt the chocolate, pour 2 inches of water into a small saucepan. Place a heat-safe shallow bowl overtop, ensuring the bottom is not touching the water. Add the chocolate chips and oil. Turn the heat to medium-low and, using a rubber spatula, stir the chocolate and oil until they're melted and smooth. Carefully remove from the heat.

4   Pour the melted chocolate over the walnut crust and smooth it out with a spoon so it covers the crust evenly. Place it in the fridge for 30 minutes or until firm. Remove from the fridge and sprinkle with the flakey sea salt.

5   Slice into thin bars. Store the bars in an airtight container; they will last for up to 1 week in the fridge and for up to 3 months in the freezer.

NOTE: *If these bars are left at room temperature for too long, they will start to melt!*

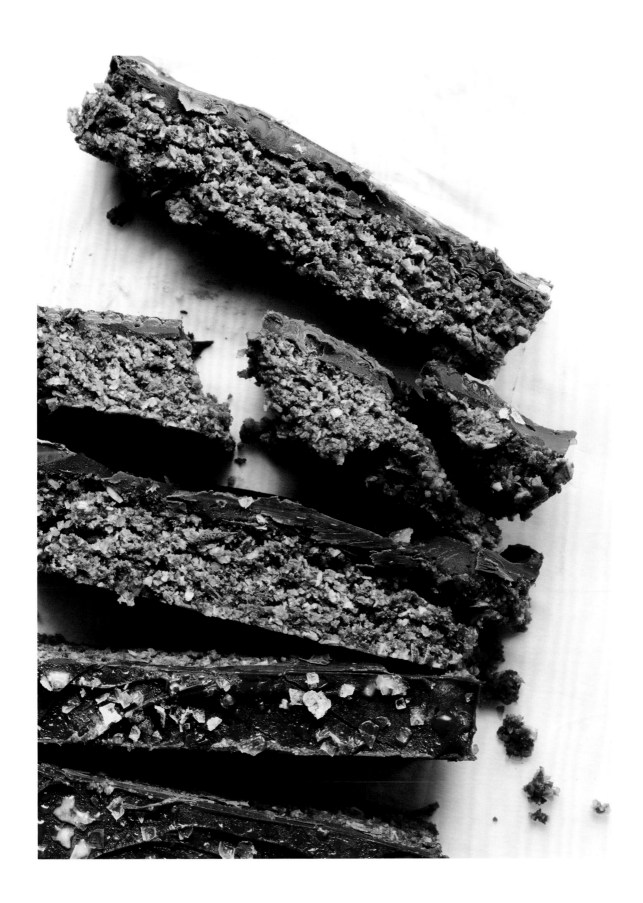

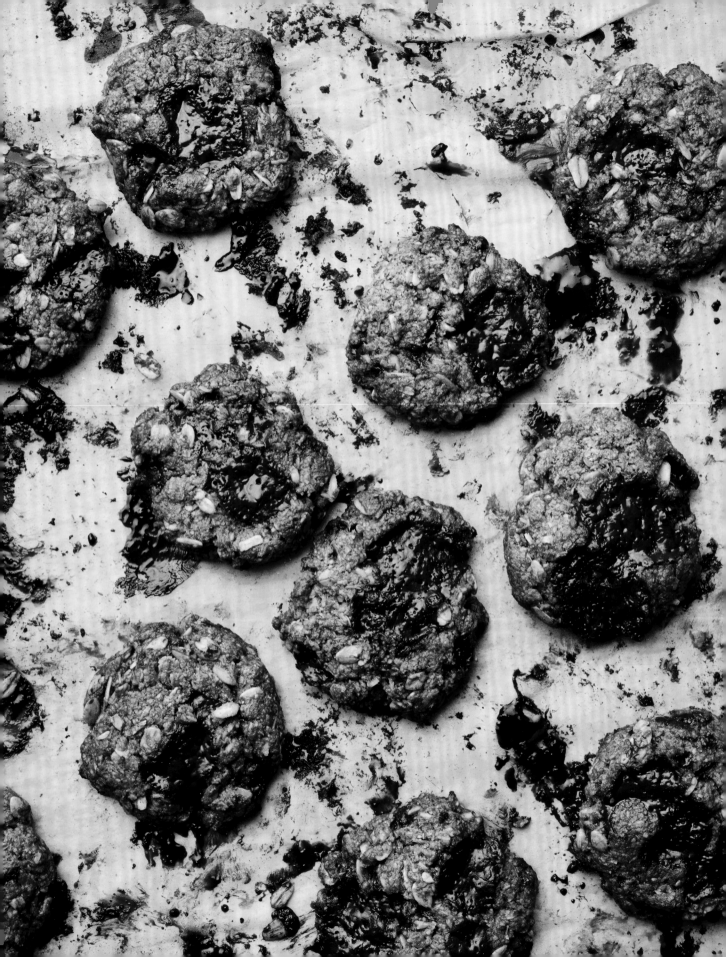

Chocolate Chunk Miso Oat Cookies

⊕ CALM, UPLIFT

PREP TIME: 10 MINUTES **BAKE TIME:** 14 MINUTES **MAKES:** 14 COOKIES

1 Tbsp ground flaxseed

3 Tbsp water

⅓ cup coconut sugar

¼ cup melted and cooled coconut oil or unsalted butter

2 Tbsp white miso paste

¾ cup oat flour

½ cup rolled oats

½ cup unsweetened shredded coconut

½ tsp baking soda

¼ tsp sea salt

½ cup roughly chopped dark chocolate bar

We added our fermented friend, miso, to these delicious cookies, which may seem odd given its salty, umami flavor. However, the savory, sweet, salty, and fatty components of these cookies all blend together so wonderfully, even the skeptics will fall in love with them. The cookies are full of fiber from the flax, oats, and coconut—this means you can avoid the post-cookie crash and remain satisfied and energized after eating them.

1 Preheat the oven to 350°F and line a baking sheet with parchment paper.

2 Combine the ground flaxseed with the water in a large bowl and let it stand for 5 minutes.

3 Mix the coconut sugar, oil, and miso into the flaxseed to get a smooth, creamy mixture. Add the oat flour, oats, coconut, baking soda, and salt and stir to combine into cookie dough. Fold in the chocolate.

4 Using your hands, roll out 1 Tbsp of cookie dough, place it on the prepared baking sheet, and gently flatten (see note). Repeat with the remaining dough, ensuring each cookie is spaced about 2-inches apart on the sheet.

5 Bake for 10–12 minutes, until the tops start to brown lightly and the edges are slightly crisp. Allow to cool on the baking sheet for 10 minutes—this helps the cookies solidify—before digging in. Store leftovers in an airtight container at room temperature for up to 2 days and then in the fridge for up to 4 days.

NOTES: 1. *A quick trick for making perfectly round cookies: once your cookie is flattened, place the open end of a drinking glass over the cookie and spin it around the cookie to smooth out its edges.* **2.** *You can replace the flax egg with an egg.*

Walnut Banana Bread

⊕ **CALM, FOCUS, UPLIFT**

PREP TIME: 15 MINUTES   **COOK TIME:** 45 MINUTES   **SERVES:** 8

2 large very ripe bananas

2 eggs

¼ cup coconut sugar

¼ cup melted and cooled coconut oil

1 tsp pure vanilla extract

1¼ cups almond flour

½ cup oat flour

¼ cup arrowroot starch or tapioca starch

2 tsp baking powder

½ tsp sea salt

½ cup roughly chopped walnuts

Sarah: This is the banana bread my husband makes for us every few weeks—(1) because we love it, and (2) because the act of baking is relaxing and helps him feel less stressed. We both love having a healthy baked good in the house, and we usually end up with some very ripe bananas lying around, which are needed for this recipe. You'll find this banana bread is high in protein and healthy fat, thanks to the almond flour, eggs, coconut oil, and walnuts, and we use only a small amount of low-glycemic coconut sugar, to enhance the natural sweetness of the bananas. The combination of these ingredients makes for a treat that's less likely to lead to a blood sugar spike and crash and instead leaves you feeling alert, energized, and steady.

1   Preheat the oven to 350°F and line a 10- × 5-inch loaf pan with parchment paper.

2   Mash the bananas in a large bowl, and then whisk in the eggs, coconut sugar, oil, and vanilla until you have a nice smooth mixture.

3   Stir together the almond flour, oat flour, arrowroot starch, baking powder, and salt in another large bowl. Fold the dry ingredients into the wet ingredients until it's a smooth batter. Gently stir the walnuts into the batter, reserving some to scatter on top.

4   Pour the batter into the prepared loaf pan and scatter the reserved walnuts overtop. Bake for 45 minutes or until a toothpick or knife inserted in the center comes out clean. The top should be lightly browned. You can store the bread in an airtight container at room temperature for 1 day and then store in the fridge for up to 5 days.

NOTE: *When baking with gluten-free flours on their own, baked goods can be quite heavy and dense. Adding tapioca starch or arrowroot starch helps make gluten-free baked goods fluffier and lighter.*

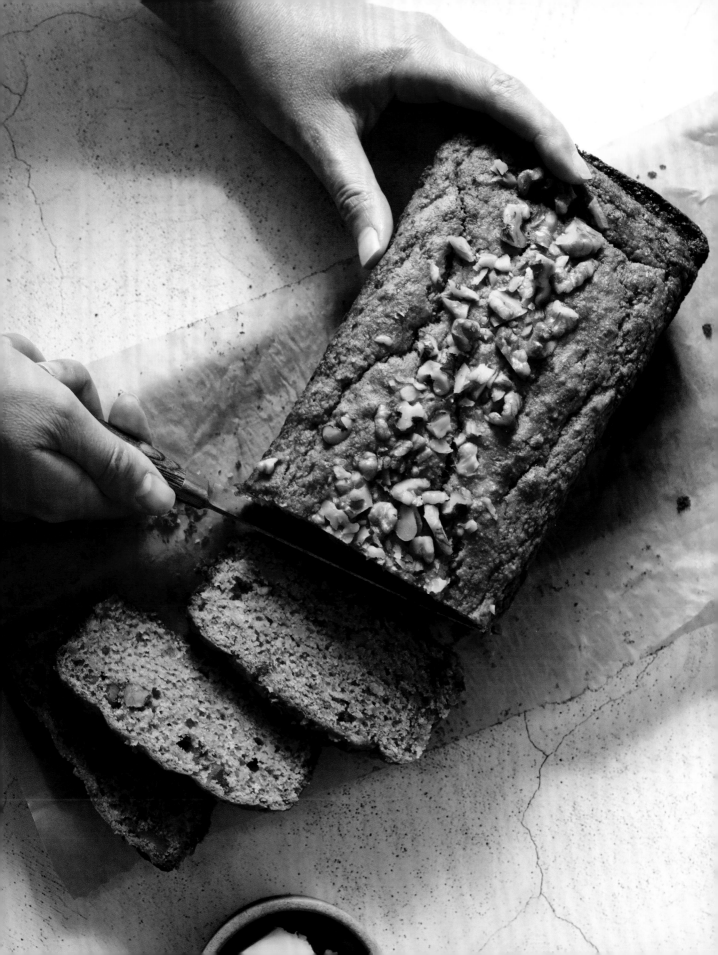

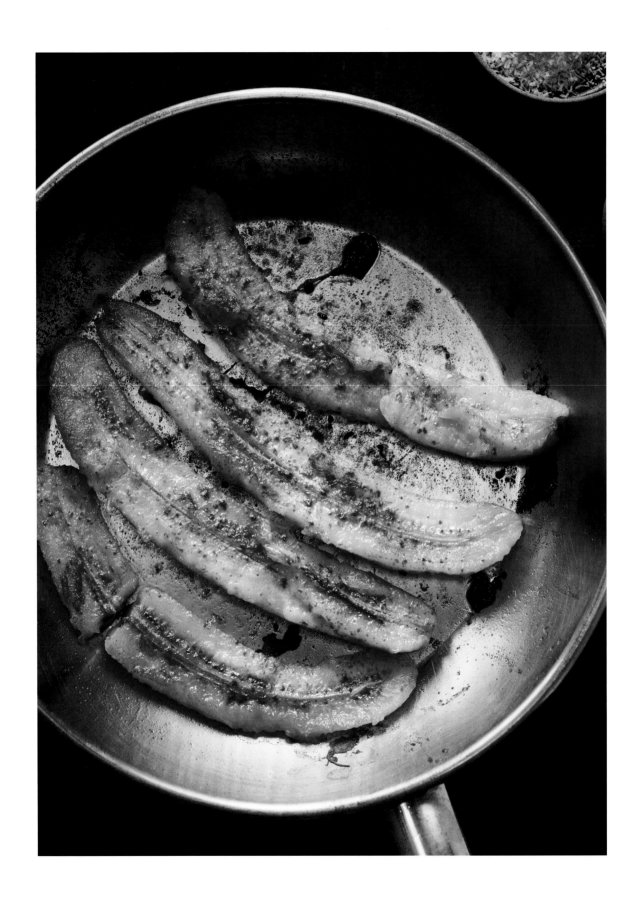

Coconut Fried Green Bananas

+ Fiber-Rich + Healthy Fats
+ Prebiotic

⊕ CALM, UPLIFT
PREP TIME: 2 MINUTES **COOK TIME:** 5 MINUTES **SERVES:** 2

2 green (unripe) bananas

1 Tbsp coconut oil

½ tsp ground cinnamon, divided

¼ cup plain yogurt, for garnish (optional)

Coconut whipped cream, for garnish (optional)

2 Tbsp unsweetened shredded coconut, lightly toasted, for garnish (optional)

1 Tbsp cacao nibs, for garnish (optional)

Drizzle of honey, for garnish (optional)

If you've ever been waiting on green bananas to ripen, wait no more! Now you can use them in this delicious dessert. It's super easy, and the green bananas will offer you a dose of prebiotics—the ones that fuel the good probiotics in your gut to help support immunity and build the feel-good neurotransmitters that support joy and pleasure. Coconut oil is a healthy and tasty oil, delicious when paired with caramelized banana and cinnamon.

1 Peel the bananas (you may need to cut the peel with a knife, if the bananas are very green) and slice in half lengthwise. If the bananas are very long, you can cut them in half horizontally as well, so you end up with 4 pieces from each banana.

2 Heat the oil in a large stainless steel skillet set over medium heat. Carefully place the bananas flat side down in the hot oil. Sear for 2 minutes, until the bananas start to brown on the bottom. Sprinkle ¼ tsp of cinnamon overtop and then flip each piece to sear the second side, for another 2 minutes. The edges will look caramelized. Sprinkle the remaining ¼ tsp cinnamon overtop.

3 Serve right away, topped with yogurt or coconut whipped cream, if you like. Sprinkle the shredded coconut and cacao nibs overtop, and add a drizzle of honey too, if you like.

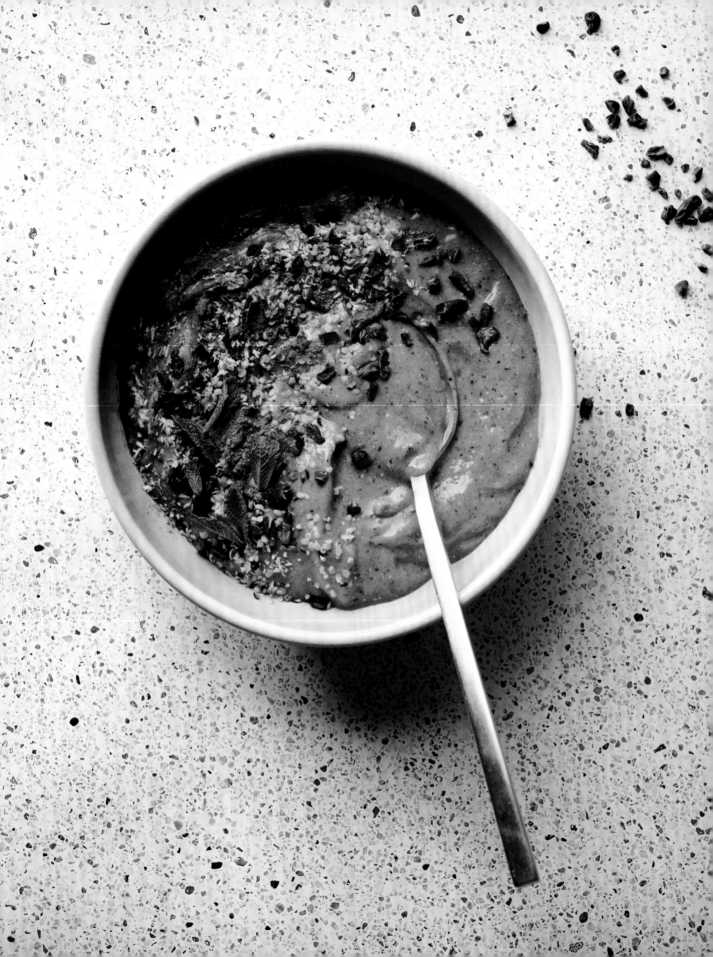

drinks

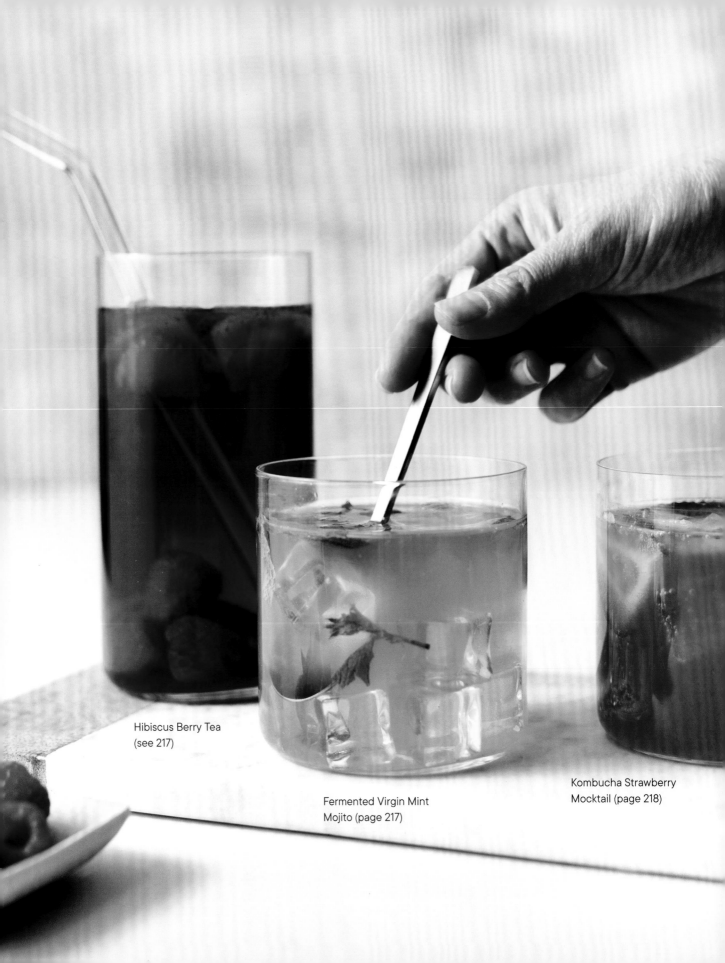

Hibiscus Berry Tea
(see 217)

Fermented Virgin Mint
Mojito (page 217)

Kombucha Strawberry
Mocktail (page 218)

Hibiscus Berry Tea

⊕ CALM, UPLIFT
PREP TIME: 10 MINUTES **SERVES:** 2

This iced tea is a beautiful, vibrant pink-red that reminds us of a tropical sunset—it makes us feel happier just sipping it. We like to add fresh berries (or frozen berries) to iced tea because they add extra flavor, a little bit of natural sweetness, and healthful polyphenols (responsible for the beautiful color of this tea) that have been found to help ease symptoms of depression and anxiety.

2 hibiscus tea bags or 1 Tbsp loose-leaf hibiscus tea

1 cup boiling water

¼ cup sliced strawberries

¼ cup raspberries

1 Tbsp freshly squeezed lemon juice

2 cups cold water

Ice

1 Place the tea in a large mug and pour the boiling water overtop. Steep for 5 minutes. Once the tea has steeped, squeeze and discard the tea bags.

2 Place the berries and lemon juice in a 2-pint mason jar. Pour in the steeped tea and the cold water.

3 You can place the jar in the fridge to cool down completely or add ice to two glasses and pour the tea overtop to cool it down. Store in an airtight container in the fridge for up to 4 days.

Fermented Virgin Mint Mojito

⊕ CALM, UPLIFT
PREP TIME: 5 MINUTES **SERVES:** 2

There's nothing like a mojito to make you feel like you're on vacation. Instead of club soda, probiotic-rich kombucha provides the fizziness, and you'll also enjoy the bite from the fermented tea. The tea helps support a healthy gut microbiome, which helps lower inflammation, ease feelings of depression, and contributes to overall mental wellness.

3 tsp coconut sugar, divided

12 fresh mint leaves, divided, plus more for garnish

Juice of 1 lime, divided

Ice

2 cups ginger kombucha, divided

NOTE: *Look for a brand of kombucha that is low in sugar on the nutrition facts label and choose any flavor of kombucha you like.*

1 Place two glasses on the counter and add 1½ tsp of coconut sugar and 6 mint leaves to each glass. Muddle the mint leaves for 30 seconds, until their fresh aroma releases and they start to break into smaller pieces. Divide the lime juice between the glasses.

2 Fill the glasses almost to the top with ice. Pour 1 cup of kombucha into each glass, stir, and garnish with mint leaves.

Kombucha Strawberry Mocktail

⊕ CALM, UPLIFT

PREP TIME: 5 MINUTES **SERVES:** 2

½ cup sliced strawberries, divided

Ice

1 cup ginger kombucha, divided

1 cup coconut water, divided

3 tsp freshly squeezed lemon juice, divided

2 strawberries, for garnish

Relax, put your feet up, and sip on this uplifting glass of bubbly! The fizzy and tart fermented kombucha pairs well with the naturally sweet coconut water. This fermented drink supports gut health, which helps build the body's happiness chemicals. It's also a rich source of B vitamins, helping the body process stress. Coconut water contains electrolytes, so it's wonderful when you need extra hydration.

1   Divide the strawberries between two glasses. Muddle the strawberries until they start to break down, but don't fully mash the berries—you can leave some small pieces.

2   Fill the glasses almost to the top with ice. Pour ½ cup of kombucha into each glass. Pour ½ cup of coconut water and 1½ tsp of lemon juice into each glass, and give the mixture a stir.

3   Garnish each glass with a strawberry and enjoy right away!

NOTE: *Look for a brand of kombucha that is low in sugar on the nutrition facts label. Although kombucha contains probiotics for your gut, it can trigger IBS symptoms, so if you know this is a trigger food for you, use coconut water instead of kombucha.*

Mood-Boosting Mocha Smoothie

½ cup brewed and cooled coffee
  (decaf or caffeinated, see note)

½ cup milk of choice

4 frozen cauliflower florets

½ banana or 2 pitted dates

1 Tbsp natural almond butter

1 heaping Tbsp cacao powder or
  cocoa powder

1 scoop of protein powder of
  choice (chocolate variety
  would be best!)

⊕ **ENERGIZE, FOCUS, UPLIFT**

PREP TIME: 5 MINUTES **SERVES:** 1

Chocolate and coffee are a perfect pair—so why not put them together in a smoothie that supports your brain *and* tastes like a dessert? The frozen cauliflower florets do double duty, acting like ice cubes while also adding fiber and antioxidants. Cacao, protein, and almond butter all have unique mood-boosting ingredients, which help relieve stress, create steady energy, and support memory.

1   If you have a high-speed blender, toss everything in and blend until smooth. If you don't, blend the coffee, milk, and cauliflower until smooth, then add the banana, almond butter, cacao powder, and protein powder. Blend until smooth.

NOTE: *We prefer using decaf coffee, but you can use regular if you're looking for that hit of caffeine.*

½ tsp grated ginger

1 cup loosely packed baby
   spinach or green kale

4 frozen cauliflower florets or
   ¼ cup frozen zucchini

½ cup unsweetened kefir,
   yogurt, or dairy-free yogurt

½ cup milk of choice

½ cup mango (fresh or frozen)

1 Tbsp hemp seeds

1 tsp chia seeds or flaxseed

1 scoop vanilla or unflavored
   protein powder

Ginger Greens Smoothie

⊕ ENERGIZE, UPLIFT

PREP TIME: 5 MINUTES **SERVES:** 1

We love a green smoothie option that everyone will enjoy—kids included! If you ever have a day where you didn't get to eat a lot of veggies, drink this smoothie! It's easy to get a variety of produce into this smoothie so you won't miss out on fiber, polyphenols, and even B vitamins, all of which support your gut bacteria and a balanced, steady mood.

1   If you have a high-speed blender, toss everything into it and blend until smooth. Otherwise, blend the ginger, spinach, and cauliflower with the kefir and milk until smooth, then add the mango, hemp seeds, chia seeds, and protein powder. Blend until smooth.

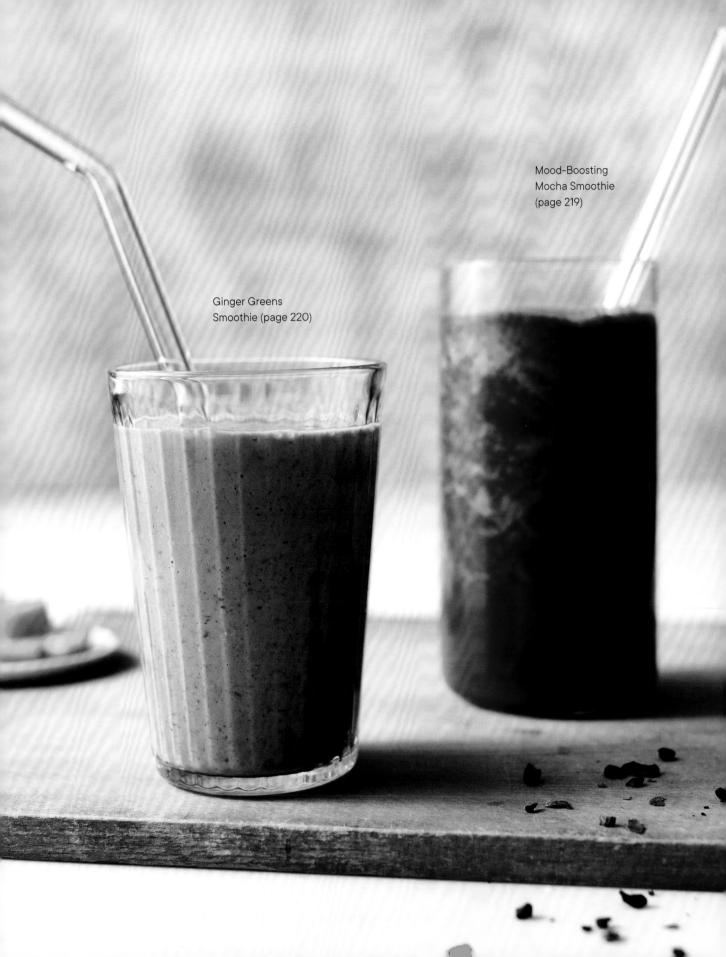

Mood-Boosting
Mocha Smoothie
(page 219)

Ginger Greens
Smoothie (page 220)

Coconut Ginger Sleepy Time Latte

⊕ CALM, SLEEP

PREP TIME: 5 MINUTES   **COOK TIME:** 5 MINUTES   **SERVES:** 1

½ cup full-fat canned coconut milk

1 cup milk of choice

1 Medjool date, pitted (see note)

1 Tbsp hemp seeds

1 tsp grated ginger

¼ tsp ground cinnamon

1 chamomile tea bag

This is the perfect drink to sip to get cozy and relaxed before bed. Chamomile is a calming herb, and we incorporate it into this creamy, frothy tea latte to help you relax at the end of the day. Hemp seeds provide some protein and healthy fat to support your blood sugar balance—which is so important for a long, restful sleep.

1   Place the coconut milk, milk, date, hemp seeds, ginger, and cinnamon in a blender and blend until smooth and creamy.

2   Pour the blended mixture into a small pot set over medium heat and heat for 5 minutes or until steaming and hot, just below boiling. Pour the mixture over the chamomile tea bag in a mug and let steep for 5 minutes before serving.

NOTE: *If you don't like or have Medjool dates, you can swap in a different type of date or use ½–1 tsp of honey instead.*

Blood Sugar Balancing Hot Chocolate

⊕ **CALM, ENERGIZE, UPLIFT**

PREP TIME: 10 MINUTES **SERVES:** 1

1½ cups milk of choice

1 large Medjool date, pitted (see note)

2 tsp cacao powder or cocoa powder

1 Tbsp hemp seeds

1 Tbsp natural almond butter

Whether it's a snow day or a dreary gray rainy day, or you just crave a comforting drink, a mug of this hot chocolate is perfect to cozy up with. Unlike packaged hot cocoa, which is typically loaded with sugar, here we use high-fiber dates for sweetness and the healthy fat and protein in hemp seeds and almond butter to keep your blood sugar steady, so you'll feel balanced and revitalized after drinking this.

1 Pour the milk into a small pot and heat over medium heat until it's about to boil. Keep an eye on the milk to make sure it doesn't scorch (you can stir every couple of minutes).

2 Once the milk is very hot, carefully pour it into a blender. Add the date, cacao powder, hemp seeds, and almond butter. Blend until smooth and creamy. Pour into a mug and enjoy right away!

NOTE: *If you don't have Medjool dates, you can use another type of date, but will probably need 2 dates if they are smaller.*

Mint Chip "Ice Cream" Smoothie Bowl

⊕ ENERGIZE, FOCUS, UPLIFT

PREP TIME: 10 MINUTES **SERVES:** 1

½ cup ripe avocado

1 heaping cup chopped frozen banana

1 cup milk of choice

½ cup loosely packed baby spinach

2 Tbsp hemp seeds

¼ tsp peppermint extract (see note)

¼ cup cacao nibs or chopped dark chocolate bar

1 tsp cacao powder, for serving (optional)

2 tsp unsweetened shredded coconut, for serving (optional)

2 tsp hemp seeds, for serving (optional)

If you love mint chocolate chip ice cream, like we do, then you definitely need this recipe in your life. It does quadruple duty as a beverage, breakfast, snack, and even dessert. This recipe is particularly loaded in fiber and healthy fats from the avocado, hemp seeds, and cacao. After eating, you'll feel perfectly satisfied and refreshed.

1   Place the avocado, banana, milk, spinach, hemp seeds, and peppermint extract in a high-speed blender and blend until smooth and thick.

2   If you're not working with a high-speed blender, place the avocado and frozen banana in the blender with the milk and blend. You may need to stop the motor occasionally to mix the mixture with a spoon. Add the spinach, hemp seeds, and peppermint extract and blend until the mixture is smooth and thick.

3   Pour into a big bowl and sprinkle the cacao nibs overtop. Then top with the cacao powder, coconut, and hemp seeds, if you like. Enjoy right away!

NOTE: *If you love peppermint and prefer a stronger taste, add ½ tsp of peppermint extract.*

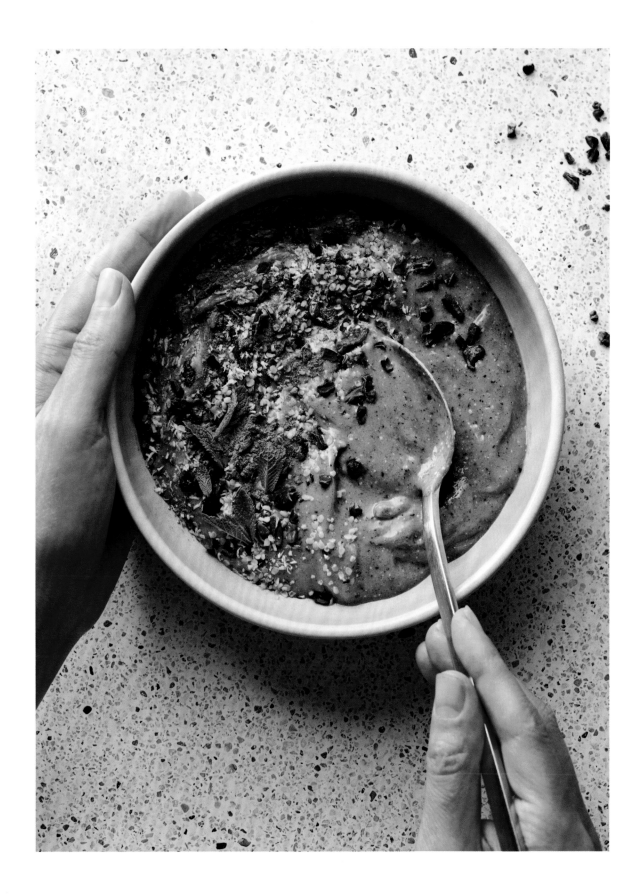

Endnotes

1   World Health Organization (2021, September 13), *Depression*, who.int/news-room/fact-sheets /detail/depression; ADAA (2022, June 27), *Anxiety Disorders—Facts & Statistics,* adaa.org /understanding-anxiety/facts-statistics.

2   American Psychological Association (2020), *Stress in America™ 2020: A National Mental Health Crisis*.

3   Breit S., Kupferberg A., Rogler G., and Hasler G. (2018), Vagus nerve as modulator of the brain—gut axis in psychiatric and inflammatory disorders, *Frontiers in Psychiatry* 9(44), doi: 10.3389/fpsyt.2018.00044.

4   Irving, P., Barrett, K., Nijher, M., and de Lusignan, S. (2021), Prevalence of depression and anxiety in people with inflammatory bowel disease and associated healthcare use: population-based cohort study, *Evidence-Based Mental Health*, doi.org/10.1136/ebmental -2020-300223; Clapp, M., Aurora, N., Herrera, L., Bhatia, M., Wilen, E., and Wakefield, S. (2017), Gut microbiota's effect on mental health: the gut-brain axis, *Clinics and Practice* 7(4), doi.org/10.4081/cp.2017.987.

5   Limbana, T., Khan, F., and Eskander, N. (2020), Gut microbiome and depression: how microbes affect the way we think, *Cureus*, doi.org/10.7759/cureus.9966.

6   Enders, Giulia (2018), *Gut: The Inside Story of Our Body's Most Underrated Organ*, Greystone Books.

7   Clapp et al., *Clinics and Practice* 7(4); Silva Y.P., Bernardi, A., and Frozza, R.L. (2020), The role of short-chain fatty acids from gut microbiota in gut-brain communication, *Front. Endocrinol.* 11(25), doi: 10.3389/fendo.2020.00025.

8   Fülling, C., Dinan, T.G., and Cryan, J.F. (2019), Gut microbe to brain signaling: what happens in vagus. . . . *Neuron* 101(6), 998–1002, doi.org/10.1016/j.neuron.2019.02.008.

9   Radjabzadeh, D., Bosch, J.A., Uitterlinden, A.G., et al. (2022), Gut microbiome-wide association study of depressive symptoms, *Nature Communications* 13(1), 7128, doi.org/10.1038/s41467 -022-34502-3.

10 McDonald, D., Hyde, E., Debelius, J.W., Morton, J.T., Gonzalez, A., Ackermann, G., Aksenov, A.A., Behsaz, B., Brennan, C., Chen, Y., DeRight Goldasich, L., Dorrestein, P.C., Dunn, R.R., Fahimipour, A.K., Gaffney, J., Gilbert, J.A., Gogul, G., Green, J.L., Hugenholtz, P., and Humphrey, G. (2018), American gut: an open platform for citizen science microbiome research, *mSystems* 3(3), doi.org/10.1128/msystems.00031-18.

11 McDonald et al., *mSystems* 3(3).

12 Valles-Colomer, M., Falony, G., Darzi, Y., Tigchelaar, E.F., Wang, J., Tito, R.Y., Schiweck, C., Kurilshikov, A., Joossens, M., Wijmenga, C., Claes, S., Van Oudenhove, L., Zhernakova, A., Vieira-Silva, S., and Raes, J. (2019), The neuroactive potential of the human gut microbiota

in quality of life and depression, *Nature Microbiology* 4(4), 623–32, doi.org/10.1038/s41564-018-0337-x.

13 Carabotti, M., Scirocco, A., Maselli, M.A., and Severi, C. (2015), The gut-brain axis: interactions between enteric microbiota, central and enteric nervous systems, *Annals of Gastroenterology* 28(2), 203–09, ncbi.nlm.nih.gov/pmc/articles/PMC4367209/.

14 Oliver, A., Chase, A.B., Weihe, C., Orchanian, S.B., Riedel, S.F., Hendrickson, C.L., Lay, M., Sewall, J.M., Martiny, J.B.H., and Whiteson, K. (2021), High-fiber, whole-food dietary intervention alters the human gut microbiome but not fecal short-chain fatty acids, *mSystems* 6(2), doi.org/10.1128/msystems.00115–21.

15 McDonald et al., *mSystems* 3(3).

16 Wastyk, H., Fragiadakis, G., Perelman, D., Dahan D., Merrill B., Yu, F., Topf, M., Gonzalez, C., Treuren, W., Han, S., Robinson, J., Elias, J., Sonnenburg, E., Gardner, C., et al. (2021), Gut-microbiota-targeted diets modulate human immune status, *Cell*, doi.org/10.1016/j.cell.2021.06.019.

17 Chao, L., Liu, C., Sutthawongwadee, S., Li, Y., Lv, W., Chen, W., Yu, L., Zhou, J., Guo, A., Li, Z., and Guo, S. (2020), Effects of probiotics on depressive or anxiety variables in healthy participants under stress conditions or with a depressive or anxiety diagnosis: a meta-analysis of randomized controlled trials, *Frontiers in Neurology* 11, doi.org/10.3389/fneur.2020.00421.

18 Slavin, J. (2013), Fiber and prebiotics: mechanisms and health benefits, *Nutrients* 5(4), 1417–35, doi.org/10.3390/nu5041417.

19 Carlson, J.L., Erickson, J.M., Lloyd, B.B., and Slavin, J.L. (2018), Health effects and sources of prebiotic dietary fiber, *Current Developments in Nutrition* 2(3), doi.org/10.1093/cdn/nzy005.

20 Enders, *Gut*.

21 Ganesan, K., and Xu, B. (2017), A critical review on polyphenols and health benefits of black soybeans, *Nutrients* 9(5), 455, doi.org/10.3390/nu9050455.

22 Cory, H., Passarelli, S., Szeto, J., Tamez, M., and Mattei, J. (2018), The role of polyphenols in human health and food systems: a mini-review, *Frontiers in Nutrition* 5(87), doi.org/10.3389/fnut.2018.00087; Lin, K., Li, Y., Toit, E., Wendt, L., Sun, J. (2021), Effects of polyphenol supplementations on improving depression, anxiety, and quality of life in patients with depression, *Frontiers in Psychiatry* 12, frontiersin.org/articles/10.3389/fpsyt.2021.765485.

23 Nazzaro, F., Fratianni, F., De Feo, V., Battistelli, A., Da Cruz, A.G., and Coppola, R. (2020), Polyphenols, the new frontiers of prebiotics, *Advances in Food and Nutrition Research*, 94, 35–89, doi.org/10.1016/bs.afnr.2020.06.002.

24 University of Warwick (2016, July 10), Fruit and veggies give you the feel-good factor, *ScienceDaily*, sciencedaily.com/releases/2016/07/160710094239.htm.

25 Sartori, S.B., Whittle, N., Hetzenauer, A., and Singewald, N. (2012), Magnesium deficiency induces anxiety and HPA axis dysregulation: modulation by therapeutic drug treatment, *Neuropharmacology* 62(1), 304–12, doi.org/10.1016/j.neuropharm.2011.07.027; Djokic, G., Vojvodić, P., Korcok, D., Agic, A., Rankovic, A., Djordjevic, V., Vojvodic, A., Vlaskovic-Jovicevic, T., Peric-Hajzler, Z., Matovic, D., Vojvodic, J., Sijan, G., Wollina, U., Tirant, M., Thuong, N.V., Fioranelli, M., and Lotti, T. (2019), The effects of magnesium—melatonin—vit B complex supplementation in treatment of insomnia, *Open Access Macedonian Journal of Medical Sciences* 7(18), 3101–05, doi.org/10.3889/oamjms.2019.771; Boyle, N., Lawton, C., and Dye, L. (2017), The effects of magnesium supplementation on subjective anxiety and stress—a systematic review, *Nutrients* 9(5), 429, doi.org/10.3390/nu9050429; Tarleton, E.K., Littenberg, B., MacLean, C.D., Kennedy, A.G., and Daley, C. (2017), Role of magnesium supplementation in the treatment of depression: a randomized clinical trial, *PloS one* 12(6), e0180067, doi.org/10.1371/journal.pone.0180067.

26 Djokic et al., *Open Access Macedonian Journal of Medical Sciences* 7(18), 3101–05; Boyle, Lawton, and Dye, *Nutrients* 9(5), 429.

27 Kirkland, A., Sarlo, G., and Holton, K. (2018), The role of magnesium in neurological disorders, *Nutrients* 10(6), 730, doi.org/10.3390/nu10060730.

28 Sartori et al., *Neuropharmacology* 62(1), 304–12; Djokic et al., *Open Access Macedonian Journal of Medical Sciences* 7(18), 3101–05; Boyle, Lawton, and Dye, *Nutrients* 9(5), 429.

29 Pickering, G., Mazur, A., Trousselard, M., Bienkowski, P., Yaltsewa, N., Amessou, M., Noah, L., and Pouteau, E. (2020), Magnesium status and stress: the vicious circle concept revisited, *Nutrients*, *12*(12), 3672, doi.org/10.3390/nu12123672.

30 Cleveland Clinic (2014), Magnesium-rich food information, Cleveland Clinic, my.clevelandclinic.org/health/articles/15650-magnesium-rich-food.

31 Ebrahimi, E., Khayati Motlagh, S., Nemati, S., and Tavakoli, Z. (2012), Effects of magnesium and vitamin B_6 on the severity of premenstrual syndrome symptoms, *Journal of Caring Sciences* 1(4), 183–89, doi.org/10.5681/jcs.2012.026.

32 Ebrahimi et al., *Journal of Caring Sciences* 1(4), 183–89.

33 Kafeshani, M., Feizi, A., Esmaillzadeh, A., Keshteli, A.H., Afshar, H., Roohafza, H., and Adibi, P. (2020), Higher vitamin B_6 intake is associated with lower depression and anxiety risk in women but not in men: a large cross-sectional study, *International Journal for Vitamin and Nutrition Research* 90(5–6), 484–92, doi.org/10.1024/0300-9831/a000589.

34 Young, S.N. (2007), Folate and depression—a neglected problem, *Journal of Psychiatry & Neuroscience* 32(2), 80–82.

35 Sangle, P., Sandhu, O., Aftab, Z., Anthony, A T., and Khan, S. (2020), Vitamin B_{12} supplementation: preventing onset and improving prognosis of depression, *Cureus* 12(10), doi.org/10.7759/cureus.11169.

36 Kafeshani et al., *International Journal for Vitamin and Nutrition Research*, 90(5–6), 484–92.

37 Gracious, B.L., Finucane, T.L., Friedman-Campbell, M., Messing, S., and Parkhurst, M.N. (2012), Vitamin D deficiency and psychotic features in mentally ill adolescents: a cross-sectional study, *BMC Psychiatry* 12(1), doi.org/10.1186/1471–244x-12–38; Williams, J.A., Romero, V.C., Clinton, C.M., Vazquez, D.M., Marcus, S.M., Chilimigras, J.L., Hamilton, S.E., Allbaugh, L.J., Vahratian, A.M., Schrader, R.M., and Mozurkewich, E.L. (2016), Vitamin D levels and perinatal depressive symptoms in women at risk: a secondary analysis of the mothers, omega-3, and mental health study, *BMC Pregnancy and Childbirth* 16(1), doi.org/10.1186/s12884-016-0988-7.

38 Spedding S. (2014), Vitamin D and depression: a systematic review and meta-analysis comparing studies with and without biological flaws, *Nutrients* 6(4), 1501–18, doi.org/10.3390/nu6041501.

39 Liao, Y., Xie, B., Zhang, H., He, Q., Guo, L., Subramaniapillai, M., Fan, B., Lu, C., and Mclntyer, R.S. (2019), Efficacy of omega-3 PUFAs in depression: a meta-analysis, *Translational Psychiatry* 9(1), doi.org/10.1038/s41398-019-0515-5.

40 Cutuli, D. (2017), Functional and structural benefits induced by omega-3 polyunsaturated fatty acids during aging, *Current Neuropharmacology* 15(4), 534–42, doi.org/10.2174/1570159x14666160614091311.

41 Stahl, L.A., Begg, D.P., Weisinger, R.S., and Sinclair, A.J. (2008), The role of omega-3 fatty acids in mood disorders, *Current Opinion in Investigational Drugs* 9(1), 57–64, pubmed.ncbi.nlm.nih.gov/18183532/; Yehuda, S., Rabinovitz, S., and Mostofsky, D.I. (2005), Mixture of essential fatty acids lowers test anxiety, *Nutr. Neurosci.* 8, 265–67, tandfonline.com/doi/abs/10.1080/10284150500445795.

42 Larrieu, T., and Layé, S. (2018), Food for mood: relevance of nutritional omega-3 fatty acids for depression and anxiety. *Frontiers in Physiology* 9, 1047, doi.org/10.3389/fphys.2018.01047.

43 Patterson, E., Wall, R., Fitzgerald, G.F., Ross, R.P., and Stanton, C. (2012), Health implications of high dietary omega-6 polyunsaturated fatty acids, *Journal of Nutrition and Metabolism* 2012, 539426, doi.org/10.1155/2012/539426.

44 Larrieu and Layé, *Frontiers in Physiology* 9, 1047.

45 Harvard T.H. Chan (2019, May 22), Omega-3 fatty acids: an essential contribution, The Nutrition Source, hsph.harvard.edu/nutritionsource/what-should-you-eat/fats-and-cholesterol/types-of-fat/omega-3-fats/.

46 National Institutes of Health (2017), Office of Dietary Supplements—Omega-3 Fatty Acids, Nih.gov, ods.od.nih.gov/factsheets/Omega3FattyAcids-Consumer/.

47 U.S. Department of Health and Human Services and U.S. Department of Agriculture (2015), *2015–2020 Dietary Guidelines for Americans*, 8th ed., health.gov/dietaryguidelines/2015/guidelines/.

48 National Institute of Health (2017), Office of Dietary Supplements—Omega-3 Fatty Acids, Nih.gov, ods.od.nih.gov/factsheets/Omega3FattyAcids-HealthProfessional/.

49 National Institute of Health (2017), Office of Dietary Supplements—Omega-3 Fatty Acids, Nih.gov, ods.od.nih.gov/factsheets/Omega3FattyAcids-HealthProfessional/; Rodriguez-Leyva, D., and Pierce, G.N. (2010), The cardiac and haemostatic effects of dietary hempseed, *Nutrition & Metabolism* 7(32), doi.org/10.1186/1743-7075-7-32; *FoodData Central* (2019), Usda.gov, fdc.nal.usda.gov/fdc-app.html#/food-details/170148/nutrients.

50 Nutt, D.J. (2008), Relationship of neurotransmitters to the symptoms of major depressive disorder, *Journal of Clinical Psychiatry* 69 Suppl E1, 4–7, pubmed.ncbi.nlm.nih.gov/18494537/.

51 Yong, S.J., Tong, T., Chew, J., and Lim, W.L. (2020), Antidepressive mechanisms of probiotics and their therapeutic potential, *Frontiers in Neuroscience* 13, doi.org/10.3389/fnins.2019.01361; Perlmutter, D. (2017), *Brain Maker: The Power of Gut Microbes to Heal and Protect Your Brain—for Life*, Yellow Kite.

52 Lydiard, R.B. (2003), The role of GABA in anxiety disorders, *Journal of Clinical Psychiatry*, 64 Suppl 3, 21–27, pubmed.ncbi.nlm.nih.gov/12662130/.

53 Jenkins, T., Nguyen, J., Polglaze, K., and Bertrand, P. (2016), Influence of tryptophan and serotonin on mood and cognition with a possible role of the gut-brain axis, *Nutrients* 8(1), 56, doi.org/10.3390/nu8010056.

54 Bloemendaal, M., Froböse, M.I., Wegman, J., Zandbelt, B.B., van de Rest, O., Cools, R., and Aarts, E. (2018), Neuro-cognitive effects of acute tyrosine administration on reactive and proactive response inhibition in healthy older adults, *Eneuro* 5(2), ENEURO.0035-17.2018, doi.org/10.1523/eneuro.0035-17.2018.

55 Khan, S., Waliullah, S., Godfrey, V., Khan, M.A.W., Ramachandran, R.A., Cantarel, B.L., Behrendt, C., Peng, L., Hooper, L.V., and Zaki, H. (2020), Dietary simple sugars alter microbial ecology in the gut and promote colitis in mice, *Science Translational Medicine* 12(567), 6218, doi.org/10.1126/scitranslmed.aay6218.

56 Townsend, G.E., Han, W., Schwalm, N.D., Raghavan, V., Barry, N A., Goodman, A.L., and Groisman, E.A. (2019), Dietary sugar silences a colonization factor in a mammalian gut symbiont, Proceedings of the National Academy of Sciences, 116(1), 233–38, doi.org/10.1073/pnas.1813780115.

57 Knüppel, A., Shipley, M.J., Llewellyn, C.H., and Brunner, E.J. (2017), Sugar intake from sweet food and beverages, common mental disorder and depression: prospective findings from the Whitehall II study, *Scientific Reports* 7(1), doi.org/10.1038/s41598-017-05649-7; Gangwisch, J.E., Hale, L., Garcia, L., Malaspina, D., Opler, M.G., Payne, M.E., Rossom, R.C., and Lane, D. (2015), High glycemic index diet as a risk factor for depression: analyses from the Women's Health Initiative, *American Journal of Clinical Nutrition* 102(2), 454–63, doi.org/10.3945/ajcn.114.103846; Morales, J., and Schneider, D. (2014), Hypoglycemia, *American Journal*

of Medicine 127(10), S17–S24, doi.org/10.1016/j.amjmed.2014.07.004; Hypoglycemia (low blood sugar) in people without diabetes, Michigan Medicine, (n.d.), uofmhealth.org, uofmhealth.org/health-library/rt1054.

58 Penckofer, S., Quinn, L., Byrn, M., Ferrans, C., Miller, M., and Strange, P. (2012), Does glycemic variability impact mood and quality of life? *Diabetes Technology & Therapeutics* 14(4), 303–10, doi.org/10.1089/dia.2011.0191.

59 National Institute of Diabetes and Digestive and Kidney Diseases (2018, May), *Insulin Resistance & Prediabetes*, National Institute of Diabetes and Digestive and Kidney Diseases, niddk.nih.gov/health-information/diabetes/overview/what-is-diabetes/prediabetes -insulin-resistance.

60 Watson, K.T., Simard, J.F., Henderson, V.W., Nutkiewicz, L., Lamers, F., Nasca, C., Rasgon, N., and Penninx, B.W.J.H. (2021), Incident major depressive disorder predicted by three measures of insulin resistance: a Dutch cohort study, *American Journal of Psychiatry* 178(10), 914–20, doi.org/10.1176/appi.ajp.2021.20101479.

61 Lyra e Silva, N. de M., Lam, M.P., Soares, C.N., Munoz, D.P., Milev, R., and De Felice, F.G. (2019), Insulin resistance as a shared pathogenic mechanism between depression and type 2 diabetes, *Frontiers in Psychiatry* 10, doi.org/10.3389/fpsyt.2019.00057.

62 Willmann, C., Brockmann, K., Wagner, R., Kullmann, S., Preissl, H., Schnauder, G., Maetzler, W., Gasser, T., Berg, D., Eschweiler, G.W., Metzger, F., Fallgatter, A.J., Häring, H.U., Fritsche, A., and Heni, M. (2020), Insulin sensitivity predicts cognitive decline in individuals with prediabetes, *BMJ Open Diabetes Research & Care* 8(2), e001741, doi.org/10.1136/bmjdrc-2020-001741.

63 Clear, J. (2018), *Atomic Habits: Tiny Changes, Remarkable Results*, Avery.

64 Howatson, G., Bell, P.G., Tallent, J., Middleton, B., McHugh, M.P., Ellis, J. (2012), Effect of tart cherry juice (Prunus cerasus) on melatonin levels and enhanced sleep quality, *European Journal of Nutrition* 51(8), 909–16, doi: 10.1007/s00394-011-0263-7.

Gratitude

To you, our readers, our clients, our followers, and our subscribers: Thank you! Thank you for your boundless support over the last decade. Because of you, we get to do what we love: write, cook, create, and teach. Like any book, this was a labor of love and being able to support your health (while making it a delicious journey) is the greatest gift.

Daniel Skwarna: Your photos are the heart and soul of this book. We're in awe of your talent, devotion to your craft, and commitment to what you do. Thank you for the many, many hours you've put into making this book shine.

To our Appetite Team: Robert McCullough, thank you for making us authors and opening up this world to us. Rachel Brown, thank you for saying yes and helping our vision come to life. Zoe Maslow, thank you for stepping in when we needed you and for your joyful energy. Victoria Walsh and Katherine Stopa, thank you for getting us to the finish line. Judy Phillips, thank you for your very keen eye! Talia Abramson, thank you for your beautiful design. Thank you to the entire Appetite team, we are forever grateful.

Suzanne Brandreth and Paige Sisley: We love you. We can't believe it's been 8 years since we started working together! Thank you for always cheering us on, pushing for what's best for us, and for helping us see the idea behind this book. Thank you to the entire CookeMcDermid team.

To our recipe testers: This book would be far less delicious if not for you. We are so grateful for your time, careful eye, effort, and feedback. Amanda Grant and Riley Zuckerman, thank you for being our lead recipe testers and especially for preparing extra food to be used on set. We're so thankful for your cooking, Dhivya Subramanian, Doris Romano, Emma Marshall, Gazal Amin, Katie Sullivan, Laura Fulton, Marianella Espana, Melissa Torio, Nicole Grabowski, Pat Volza, Palak Loizides, Rebecca Sutin, Renee O'shea, Robyn Polan, Sonja Seiler, Lara Rae, and Ushi Bagga.

To our photography and production team: Thank you, thank you Daniel, again, for your gorgeous food photography and direction on set. Shannon Laliberte, thank you for taking us to the Beaches at the crack of dawn, allowing the sunrise to be the backdrop of our photoshoot, and capturing our essence. To the creative, patient and talented Laura Fulton, Mykaela Erb, Renee O'Shea, and Riley Zuckerman, the photoshoot for this book simply could not have happened without you. Rayna Schwartz, thank you for your beautiful eye and helping find props to match our vision. A big thank you to Album Studios for the great space to do our photo shoots.

TG:

Jackson and Reese: Thank you for being my recipe-tasters, the messiest kitchen-helpers, and for having the most excitable and loving energy.

Bram: I love you. Thank you for watching the kids so I could write and recipe test this book!

Jillian: You are genuinely the best sister, I'm so lucky.

My parents, Lisa and Barry: This book was written during a time when you were experiencing many of the things we were writing about. I'm in awe of your deep commitment to your physical and mental health and your openness to continue to evolve and grow. You are incredible role-models and I love you.

SG:

Daniel: a huge third thank you to you, for being the most supportive and encouraging partner, I love you.

Lumi: I've loved recipe testing with you and your giggles and silliness in the kitchen make every day better. Dada and I love you.

Mom and Dad: I'm so grateful for your support, thank you for always encouraging me to do what I've wanted.

Leda: I love you, thank you for being my amazing sister for life, can't wait for more cooking and trips together!

Naomi: thank you for your support with caring for the little Lumi bird (especially when we were doing photos for this book)!

Laurie and Vanessa: Laur, how did I get so fortunate to have a forever best friend? Thank you for your check-ins to make sure we keep living the dreams we have. And Vanessa, thank you for always being there, your support means the world.

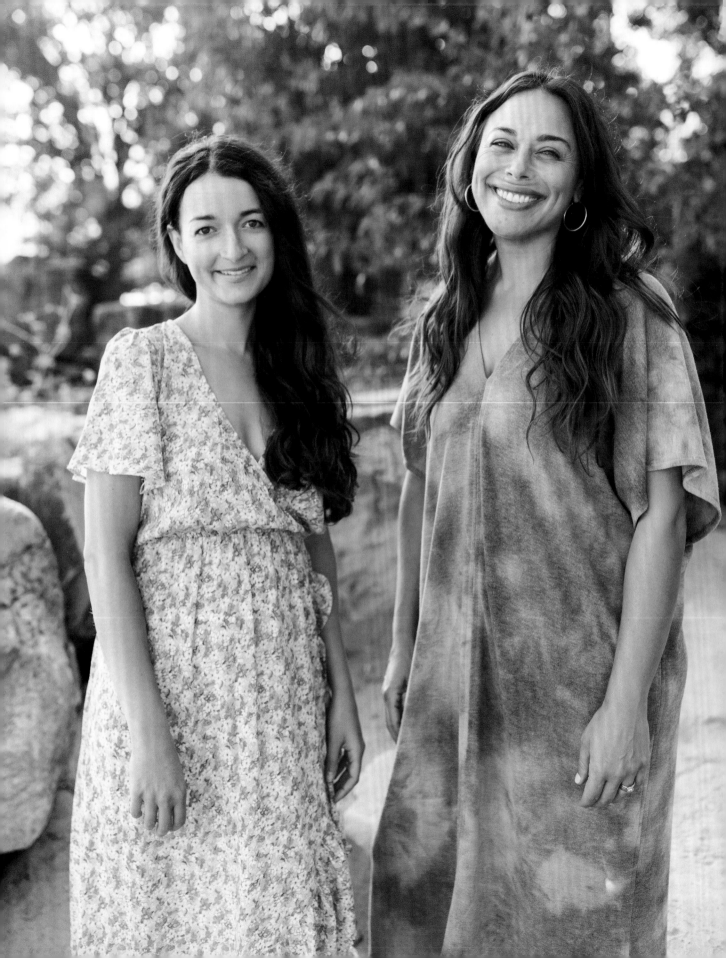

Index